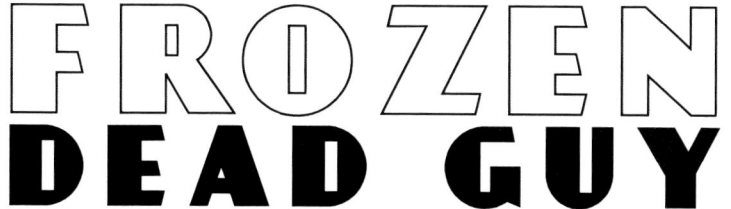

COLORADO'S ICEMAN & THE STORY OF THE
FROZEN
DEAD GUY

BO SHAFFER

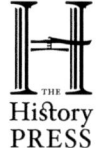

Published by The History Press
Charleston, SC 29403
www.historypress.net

Copyright © 2011 by Bo Shaffer
All rights reserved

Front cover art by Brent Warren, Imagelust Arts, www.imagelust.com.
All images are courtesy of the author.

First published 2011
Manufactured in the United States

ISBN 978.1.60949.248.9

Shaffer, Bo.
Colorado's ice man and the story of the frozen dead guy / Bo Shaffer.
p. cm.
Includes bibliographical references.
ISBN 978-1-60949-248-9
1. Shaffer, Bo. 2. Nederland (Colo.)--Biography. 3. Bauge, Trygve. 4. Morstoel, Bredo, 1900-1989. 5. Dead--Social aspects--Colorado--Nederland. 6. Cryonics--Colorado--Nederland--Case studies. 7. Ecologists--Colorado--Nederland--Biography. 8. Norwegians--Colorado--Nederland--Biography. 9. Nederland (Colo.)--Social life and customs. 10. Festivals--Colorado--Nederland. I. Title.
F784.N4S42 2011
978.8'63--dc22
2011001416

Notice: The information in this book is true and complete to the best of our knowledge. It is offered without guarantee on the part of the author or The History Press. The author and The History Press disclaim all liability in connection with the use of this book.

All rights reserved. No part of this book may be reproduced or transmitted in any form whatsoever without prior written permission from the publisher except in the case of brief quotations embodied in critical articles and reviews.

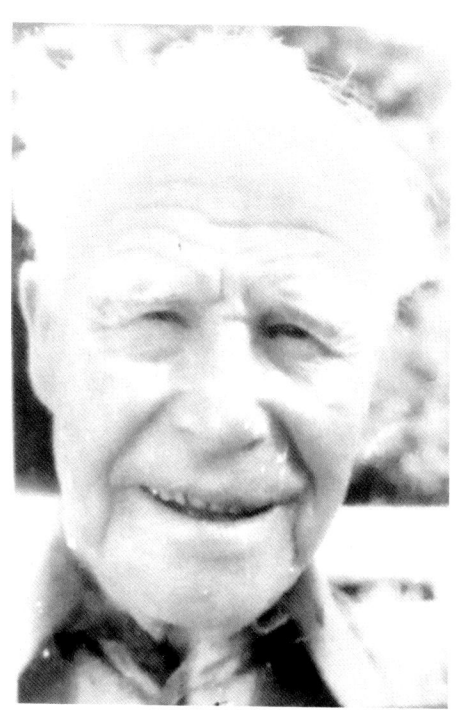

Bredo Morstoel
minor bureaucrat, father of Aud,
grandfather of Trygve,
Frozen Dead Guy.

*To my soul mate, Elizabeth, who put up with all of this.
To Morgan and Brenna, for being understanding children.*

CONTENTS

Foreword, by Marci Wheelock	11
Prologue	15
In the Beginning	17
The Iceman Cometh	23
The Early Years and the Dry Ice Wars	27
The Shed that Started It Rolling	35
Media Coverage Spreads the Word	41
Momentum Increases with the FDGD	47
The Peak Year	59
The Later Years	79
Tom Green, the Ice Hole and the Great Leno No-Show	93
Notes on Ned and the Shed	97
Psychic Phenom	109
ICICLE	115
Appendix: FAQ	121
Bibliography	125
About the Author	127

FOREWORD

Nederland is situated seventeen miles west and three thousand vertical feet up from Boulder, Colorado. By all measures, it is a small town with fewer than two thousand residents, but in no way is it an ordinary town.

Nederland is halfway between Idaho Springs and Rocky Mountain National Park on the Peak to Peak Highway, one of the most scenic drives in Colorado. On a busy summer afternoon, traffic gets jammed up around the traffic circle (we don't have a stoplight) with carloads of tourists. Nederland is known as the "Gateway to the Indian Peaks" and attracts people from all over who are looking for adventures in hiking, camping, fishing and birding. With more than fifteen feet of annual snowfall and the Eldora ski area five miles away, there is plenty to do in the winter, as well.

Nederland has endured more than its share of boom and bust cycles. In the late 1800s, gold and silver miners flocked to the area and then abruptly left when the ore from the nearby mines dried up. There was another mining boom during World War I, this time for tungsten, which was used to build battleships. Nederland's population has swelled from as many as three thousand people to as few as just a handful of hardy families able to endure the long, cold, windy winters.

Nederland has a rich musical history. There was a recording studio located at Caribou Ranch that attracted Elton John, Chicago, Michael Jackson, Tom Petty, Stephen Stills and Amy Grant to record there in the '70s and '80s. It was not uncommon to run into Dan Fogelberg or Robert Plant grabbing a beer or a burger at the Pioneer Inn. Now, Yonder

Foreword

Mountain String Band, Great American Taxi and Elephant Revival are among the successful bands that claim Nederland as home and still play at the annual NedFest and local bars.

The '60s brought the counterculture of young hippies seeking a place to drop out. In the 2010 election, voters decriminalized marijuana, and now there is a thriving medical marijuana business, bringing much-needed sales tax revenue, as well as marijuana-inspired tourism.

Today, Nederland has everything you need to lead a comfortable life: a grocery store, a hardware store, a bank, two gas stations, excellent restaurants, live music every night of the week, a movie theater, good schools and more. Still, at 8,240 feet in elevation, with breathtaking views of the Continental Divide, living here is not for the faint of heart. As some locals are fond of saying, "In Nederland, *view* is spelled w-i-n-d."

Currently, Nederland is undergoing a bit of a renaissance; it's not exactly another boom, but there is a progressive town board in place and more development than Ned has seen in a while. Amenities that make it a nice place to raise a family include a new Carousel of Happiness, an ice rink complete with curling team, a teen center, a new library, sidewalks and a skate park.

The push-pull of old-timers who would rather see things stay the same versus the newcomers who commute to Boulder for work is still present, of course, but that's another dynamic that makes our town special. A common thread that unites us all is our rugged individualism and an accepting attitude regarding our differences. There is something for everyone in Nederland.

My husband and I moved to Nederland in 2006, followed closely by our best friends and my in-laws. One thing that's great about living in a small town is how easy it is to get involved with your community. Soon after moving here, I joined the library board and then went to work for the chamber of commerce, running the Visitor's Center, and for a year now I have served on the town board.

I wonder what exactly drew Trygve Bauge to Nederland in the early '90s. He was a young man from Norway with a personal interest in cryogenics. He founded the Boulder Polar Bear Club and was known for submerging himself in freezing-cold water, all a part of his belief that ice was a means of life extension.

Trygve and his mother, Aud, began building a house on the shady side of Nederland with the intent of opening a cryogenics facility there. Aud's father, Bredo Morstoel, who died of natural causes in Norway, was already cryogenically preserved with liquid nitrogen (LN) at a facility in California.

Foreword

Once ready, they had Bredo transferred to Nederland, where they kept him frozen in a more low-tech manner, using dry ice in a shed behind their house. They also found one paying customer, Al Campbell, formerly of Chicago, for the freezing business.

Trygve was deported to Norway due to an expired visa in 1995. When Trygve was deported, Aud tipped off a reporter from the *Mountain Ear*, Nederland's local newspaper, that her dead father, along with one paying customer, was being kept frozen on their Nederland property. Soon, Aud returned to Norway also, but not before igniting an uproar.

The Nederland Police, along with the Boulder County Sherriff's Department, conducted a thorough investigation to ensure that there was no foul play. Then, the town had to figure out how to handle this bizarre discovery. At first people were outraged and even afraid that the frozen dead bodies could somehow contaminate the groundwater. Ultimately, the town board passed an ordinance making it illegal to store dead bodies within town limits, and Al Campbell was returned to his family, mostly because they were upset at the controversy. However, since Bredo had taken up residence prior to this ordinance hitting the books, he was grandfathered in and allowed to stay, thus becoming Nederland's most famous, albeit dead, resident.

It took a while for the town to settle down after the shock of learning about Grandpa. Several years later, the chamber of commerce made a bold move and hosted the first-ever Frozen Dead Guy Days in 2001. The festival, held in early March, includes a Grandpa Look-alike Contest, a parade, a Polar Plunge and Coffin Races. The festival has grown into the largest, highest-grossing event of the year in our town, bringing in more than ten thousand spectators from all over the world.

Since Trygve and Aud left town, Bo Shaffer (aka "the Iceman") has been keeping Grandpa Bredo frozen by faithfully delivering nearly two thousand pounds of dry ice to Grandpa about every four weeks, paid for by Trygve and Aud. Like Bredo Morstoel and Trygve Bauge, Bo Shaffer is also a little bit larger than life. He is hard to miss, rolling through town wearing his "I am SO Dead!" sweatshirt with a ton of dry ice loaded in his red, white and blue pickup truck decorated with political bumper stickers. He often has some strong college guy on hand to assist him unloading the ice or a news crew from another country riding shotgun. In 2008, Bo ran for Boulder County sheriff on the Libertarian ticket.

We met Bo about six weeks after moving to Nederland, when he hosted a "Grave Digger's Lunch" on Halloween. We jumped at the chance to help with an ice run and meet Bredo and Bo in person. We knew of them from

Foreword

attending Frozen Dead Guy Days and watching the documentary *Grandpa's Still in the Tuff Shed*. I must admit that I was somewhat nervous about attending a dead man's party on Halloween. Two things set me at ease: first, how seriously Bo takes his responsibilities and second, his sense of humor.

We spent about three hours with Bo and Bredo that day, and it was not creepy or scary. We had lunch in Grandpa's shed, toasted Bredo with Old Grand-Dad whiskey over dry ice and helped reload his chamber with a ton of dry ice. Bo was like a historian, sharing details of the wacky story that he had gathered in his then eleven years as Grandpa's caretaker. It occurred to me that day that Trygve had chosen the perfect person to care for his deceased, frozen grandfather.

Since then, Bo has become a good friend. He has conducted informative and entertaining tours of Grandpa's shed for our friends, Visitor's Center volunteers and even my parents from Florida. A couple years ago, he told me that other than his son I had been on more ice runs with him than anyone and that he considered me like an apprentice, in line to assume his responsibilities should he need to take a month off. If you or a loved one is ever in need of someone dependable and experienced to take care of your maintenance needs after you die, I think Bo Shaffer is your guy!

This year, 2011, marks the tenth anniversary of Frozen Dead Guy Days and will surely be the biggest and best festival to date. It is also the start of the seventeenth year that Bo Shaffer has spent dutifully taking care of keeping Bredo Morstoel frozen, making an ice run every four weeks regardless of rain, snow, shine or w-i-n-d.

–Marci Wheelock

PROLOGUE

Blow in its ear...
—Johnny Carson, on the best way to thaw a frozen turkey

Call me Iceman. This is not a name I take lightly. In my youth, I once ran up against another Iceman, who left a lasting impression on me. I was working on a project in Upstate New York, and near the end of the project we had a slight disagreement with one of our subcontractors. Now these subcontractors did not take lightly to disagreements, and in the course of my boss's conversation with their boss, there was pretty agitated talk. Well, a couple days after this talk ended, with their boss storming out of the room, I was sitting in the back room at a local bar, and a friend walks up to me and says that there was someone looking for me. Now, the nature of our business was not such that I enjoyed people looking for me at that time, so I sent them back to find out who it was. The word comes back that it's a stranger who says that he's the Iceman.

After making some very quick but appropriate inquiries in the appropriate places, I found that the Iceman was pretty much a contract enforcer from Chicago brought in by the upset boss to "explain" things to my boss, and he was looking to talk to *me*. Not being in the proper frame of mind to deal with such a thing—having spent the last few hours at the bar—and discretion being the better part of valor, I managed to slip out the back door and have the Iceman delayed long enough for me to jump in my car and get out of the parking lot before he even knew I was there. The next day, my boss, who appeared to be a little agitated, decided to settle the dispute with the

Prologue

subcontractor. When I asked him about the change of heart, he said that a very dangerous man had explained things to him in terms he could not refuse and that I should not speak of the incident anymore to anyone. When I told him of my incident in the bar the previous night, he said that I was lucky I left—the Iceman's usual technique is to eliminate an underling to impress the seriousness of the situation on the boss before negotiations begin. Not being able to find me before my boss got back to him probably saved us all a very ugly incident. I looked over my shoulder for months after that.

So to be called the Iceman brought back some bad connotations at first. But then, as I sat and thought about it, it seemed strangely appropriate. After all, I was dealing with a dead guy, even though I hadn't made him that way, and I was under contract. Every time I make an ice run with three-quarters of a ton of dry ice, people look up and say, "The Iceman cometh!" a phrase I've heard hundreds of times now. So the Iceman, caretaker of the frozen dead guy (FDG), came into being more than fifteen years ago, mostly to transport ice but also to maintain the critical cryonic chamber's temperature and stability. In those fifteen years, I've seen quite a few interesting and sometimes downright strange things. Working with cryonicists, dead bodies, drunks, government bureaucracy, deported Norwegians, psychics, spooky neighbors, festivals and international media, to name just a few, makes for memorable times and hopefully interesting reading.

I've tried to chronicle the events here in a marginally coherent fashion. You may notice a propensity to switch tenses and write as if it were the present. I tend to be time-challenged. In truth, I have a poor sense of the passage of time. In the short term, I often get caught up in things, and before I know it, hours have passed. In the long term, some things that happened last year seem like they happened ages ago, and some things from twenty years ago seem like they happened just last year. A Daytimer and a personal digital assistant (PDA) keep me on time nowadays, but it takes a lot of sorting to put together an accurate timeline.

As with all things, one's life experiences tend to color one's perception of reality. I will occasionally make forays into my personal history to try to explain my viewpoint or why things might have a special meaning (like the name Iceman). I tend to not use full names in order to protect the guilty, as well as the innocent, so often I'll refer to a helper or an associate by an initial or nickname. Then again, there are times when it's useful to know exactly who is doing what, and I'll name names.

The chronicles of the Iceman began about 1994. However, to fully understand the situation, we have to go back a bit farther.

IN THE BEGINNING

Either this man is dead, or my watch has stopped.
—Groucho Marx

It all pretty much started with an eccentric Norwegian by the name of Trygve Bauge. Trygve and his mother came to Colorado for the freedom that America offered, as well as the geography of the Rocky Mountains. The climate was very similar to that of Norway, and Trygve felt right at home with the Rocky Mountain snow and ice. He became quite interested in providing sustainable and impregnable places for people to live, work and do business, and he investigated places like civil defense shelters, old mines and underground housing. Trygve had been traveling back and forth from Norway to America for several years. A couple of times he even brought over his grandfather, Bredo Morstoel. Bredo had never set foot in Nederland but got as close as Estes Park during a couple of vacations here in America. He seemed to like it here but apparently had no desire to stay because he went back to Norway.

Now I was told that the whole family was taking a ski vacation at their chalet on the day that Bredo had his heart attack. And, of course, by the whole family I mean Bredo, Trygve and Aud. In the entire time that I've been associated with this family, I have never once heard them mention Trygve's father, or Aud's husband. Apparently he had a falling out with the family and left around the time Trygve was a teenager. I got the feeling that he was a real persona non grata with both Trygve and his mother. But I did hear once that Trygve had a sister who lives in Italy, but she apparently spends very little time with Trygve and doesn't really agree with his philosophies. In fact, once she stole Aud away from Trygve, and Trygve couldn't get any money to operate the ice run for a period of several months…but I'm getting ahead of myself.

Like I said, the whole family was there, and even though Bredo loved to ski, he was too old to really enjoy the sport anymore. But he still liked to go with the family and spend time in the snow at their private little retreat in the mountains. On this particular trip, he had turned in upon arrival, and no one thought any more about it. The next morning, they found him stone-cold dead in bed from a heart attack. According to Trygve, in his last moments Bredo had pushed his pillows together in the shape of a "T." Now, again according to Trygve, this meant that Bredo wanted Trygve to take care of him after he died. Trygve promptly decided that his grandfather should be cryonically preserved in order that someday he might be reanimated.

For those of you who might not know what "cryonics" is, I suggest you go online, Google it and read all of the fun and interesting facts. For those of you who aren't reading this with a computer or a Kindle, cryonics is the science of preserving the physical body of a human being using supercold, cryogenic temperatures and special techniques in order that, someday, advanced science might be able to reanimate the subject. Sometimes this involves curing what killed the subject, or it might involve bringing the subject back to a state before death. Now, of course, all of this really only works if you're an objectivist. An objectivist (according to Ayn Rand) is someone who believes that the soul is intimately tied to the physical body. When the physical body dies and deteriorates, the soul goes away. If you could rebuild the physical body back to the way it was, the soul would go back into the body—a very simple explanation for death. In the case of cryonics and those who believe in it, one has to wonder what the soul does in between those times. Sits around in a garage in Buffalo? I suppose details like this are not all that relevant to true cryonicists.

And so poor Bredo was hustled off to the nearest cryonics facility. Unfortunately, this was in California, as any kind of above-ground preservation of human remains was not allowed in the European Union. This is why you will find almost all of the cryonic facilities in the world located in the United States. Also a bit unfortunate is the fact that in Norway they still have laws concerning premature burial. Anyone who dies from unknown causes in Norway cannot be embalmed for a period of time ranging from twenty-four to forty-eight hours. So after sitting around a day or two in Norway, Bredo was shipped off to a facility in Los Angeles (which

In the Beginning

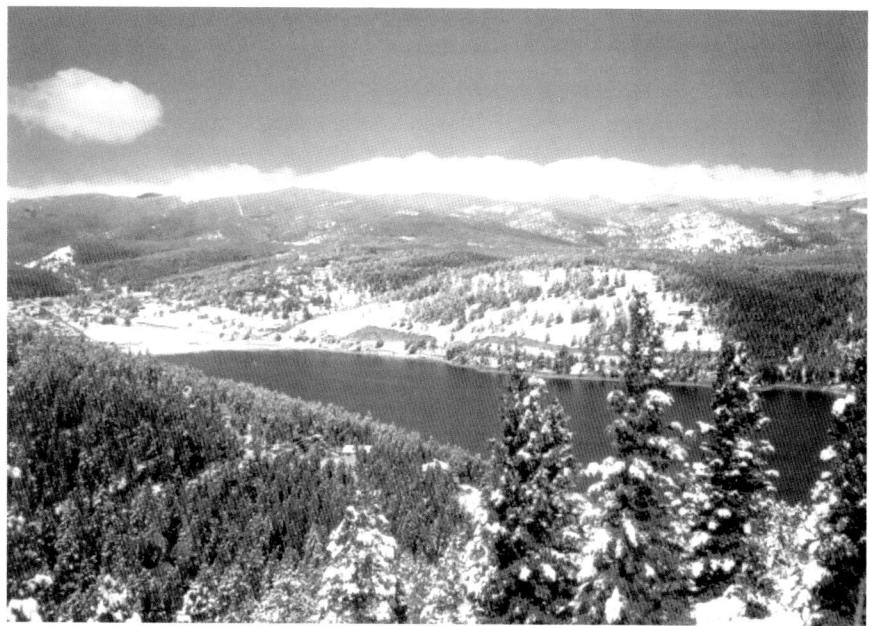

The view from the property in Nederland on one of those special winter days in Colorado.

took a day or so), where they started the process to preserve him cryonically. This also took about a day. So it took between two to four days before Bredo was fully preserved. I've seen a picture of Trygve on bended knee, like a trophy big game hunter, holding open the lid of an octagonal sarcophagus holding a very dead-looking body. (This sarcophagus appears to be the very sarcophagus in the cryonic chamber at the International Cryonics Institute where Bredo is currently kept on ice.)

Bredo died in 1989 and was kept in California for several years. During this time, Trygve finally decided to move to Colorado, buy a piece of property and build a house. The property was an outstanding piece with a magnificent view of the divide and the town of Nederland. Of course, this was not to be just any house. This house was to be earthquake-proof, bombproof and fireproof and have room for cryonically preserved body storage, as well as be sustainable and economical. In the early 1990s, Trygve secured a bank loan and started to build his dream house. One of the first things he constructed was a massive cement slab off to one side of the property. This was to be the base for the cryonic storage facility. For temporary storage, Trygve installed a couple of tin garden sheds to hold supplies and Grandpa. Sometime in late

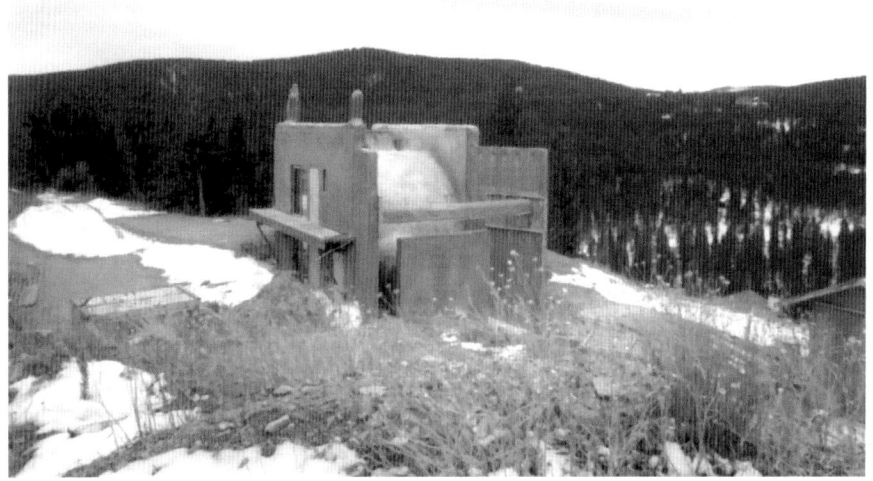

The property with the institute's main building.

1993, Trygve transported both Bredo and Bredo's roommate (more on that in just a bit) to the homemade cryonic storage box inside the little tin garden shed. Trygve had built enough of the main house to enable him and Aud to actually live there, more or less. The electricity was brought in with an extension cord from the outside panel. The water was just a stub inside the bathroom area, with no real plumbing. There was a chemical toilet outside in one of the outbuildings. The heat came solely from a small wood stove on the ground level that Aud would have to stoke every couple of hours. Trygve would stay upstairs on the heated water bed. Trygve intentionally had the only access to the second floor—a rickety old aluminum stepladder that only he could climb, effectively keeping his mother out of his "stuff."

Trygve was into more than just cryonics and life extension. He was also a dyed-in-the-wool libertarian. He firmly believed that there should be free and open borders between all countries. He taunted the Immigration and Naturalization Service (INS) incessantly for several years, trying to make his point. He hoped to force the issue that he was an illegal alien into the courts, where he would argue eloquently for the libertarian concept of free and open borders—and that he ought to be allowed to stay without his green card. Unfortunately, after being embarrassed for several years in the media, the INS decided to just grab Trygve and throw his butt on a plane back to Norway—sans court, sans hearing, sans everything—leaving his mother to fend for herself.

In the process of being interviewed over her son's deportation, Aud mentioned that she didn't know how she was going to deal with the bodies in the shed. The mere mention of bodies was enough to prick up the reporter's ears, and before you knew it the entire town was aware of what was in the sheds on the hill. There were some people in Nederland who were sure that the world would end if people started to store bodies on their property. The mayor seemed to take it as a personal affront. There were a few weeks of mass hysteria during which time an ordinance was passed essentially making it illegal for anyone to store a frozen whole body on their premises. Unfortunately, the ordinance failed to define a body as necessarily human, and thus current Nederland law prohibits frozen turkeys in freezers. Fortunately, however, Grandpa Bredo was grandfathered in. He and his roommate could stay.

Yeah, he had a roommate, Al Campbell—Big Al from Chicago, as I called him. Well, Big Al's family decided that there was too much publicity and wanted to bring Big Al back home to Chicago. Big Al definitely had the guest bed, as he was pretty much wrapped in just a sleeping bag. According to an eyewitness, it was pretty interesting to see a frozen body being moved in a sleeping bag. His family brought him back and, as far as we know, stuck him in the ground. Then Aud decided to leave. She went back to Norway after everything had settled down a little and arranged for a friend to continue with the dry ice for the cryonic storage facility.

Now we're at the spring of 1994, and Trygve's friend is getting pretty tired of transporting ice and not getting paid for it. Trygve owes him a lot of money, and he is threatening to stop transporting ice if he doesn't get paid. Trygve is desperate. One day, while posting to a futuristic mailing list called the Extropian List (this is in the days before the World Wide Web, when it was just amazing to talk to people all over the world for free using e-mails and mailing lists), someone from Colorado reads the post.

THE ICEMAN COMETH

There is no cure for birth and death, save to enjoy the interval.
—George Santayana

I was always at the forefront of technology, being a bit of a techno-geek myself. I had worked for many years as an electronic game repairman, and in college, one of my roommates was so into it that he built his own computer from scratch, including programming the machine language. When computers first came out, I would spend time in the university computer labs going "online" and playing these cool games that had few graphics (about none) and all this "interactive" maze and puzzle solving. I still remember the flowchart and the magic word "xyzzy" from *Adventure*. But all of this paled in comparison to actually having a personal computer right in my very own office. And being able to send and receive letters (more or less) instantaneously with anyone in the world who was also hooked up was cool beyond description.

I found a group called the Extropians, who were a bunch of futurists, and joined its e-mail list. Founded by Max Moore in my old stomping grounds of Santa Cruz, I was irresistibly drawn to the transhumanist movement and the possibility of making the universe a more ordered place. In the midst of several annotated conversations with these unusual minds, I came across a name I recognized. Trygve is a pretty unusual name, not unlike my own, and I had seen it in the newspapers just a few months before. So, being the friendly type and already dimly aware of a connection, I e-mailed him. "Hey, I saw your name in the papers, you used to be around here," I said to him. He responded within a few days, and we struck up a conversation. Eventually, he asked me if I wanted a job, and when I asked him, "Doing what?" he sure told me.

Now, I had just started in a new direction in my business. After graduating from University of Colorado–Boulder with a graduate degree in environmental biology, I spent several years trying to get a job in my field. Eventually, I had a three-inch stack of rejection letters, and after driving pizza delivery for both money and food (two small birds with one tiny stone), I decided that I needed to do something more substantial to support my burgeoning family.

So, being a handy sort of guy, I decided to start a construction business with a couple partners. We built the business up to the point of doing $500,000 projects, with my general contractor's license covering the company for constructing multilevel commercial buildings. I had been trying to incorporate my formal education into my vocation and started to tout my "non-toxic" construction practices and my environmental inspection abilities as things that set me apart from the rest of the pack. In fact, I had just started using the term "planetary ecologists" to describe the work we did. That term was taken from *Dune*, Frank Herbert's ecological science fiction masterpiece. I felt, just like Liet-Kynes, a deep compulsion to make the planet better for everyone. And then I got offered one of the most unusual yet intensely ecological jobs ever located in Colorado: maintaining the cryogenic temperatures in a homemade cryonic preservation chamber with no electricity in a homemade bomb shelter perched on the top of a mountain—with the future resurrection and subsequent life of a dead grandfather at stake. I had a few questions.

When I had heard all of the details, I realized that this was a bit more than I had ever contemplated, but the thought of working with an international client on a totally unique local project was irresistible to me. Trygve got me in contact with his friend who was doing the ice transportation at that time but was getting pretty tired of doing it and not getting paid. He was just about to stop buying ice (Trygve owed him more than $1,000) and was relieved that someone else had agreed to take on the incredible responsibility of seeing that Trygve's grandfather was kept in a cryonic state, ready for reanimation. In fact, it was impressed upon me at the very beginning that if I were to fail in this responsibility at any time, I would be responsible for killing Bredo. Killing a dead person…quite an interesting concept, and something over which I've spent many an hour engaged in philosophical discourse, I assure you.

In the end, I agreed to take over the ice transportation and maintenance of the facility. Trygve set me up to meet with his friend Walter. Walter is a nice guy—to a fault. People seem to sense this and have a tendency to take advantage of him. Trygve had been imposing on him and another friend the duty to maintain this facility with dry ice loads brought up every couple of weeks. They had even been using their own money until Trygve could send his own, but they were stretched to the limit covering Trygve's finances. Having a "new guy" take over the ice shipments allowed Tryg to finance a current ice carrier who wasn't upset about not being paid and hold off on reimbursing his friends for a while. Sort of like a refinancing. Eventually, Trygve paid everybody back, but at the time it was a financial breathing space.

Walter took me up to the site for the first time, and although I'm an Eagle Scout, I got a bit confused as to how to find the place. All of those forest roads look alike. Eventually, I got to the point where I could probably find the way out blindfolded in a snowstorm (I'll save that story for later), but to this day I like to occasionally let the newbies find their own way out and follow them around and around—although confusing and twisty, all of the roads in that area are loops, and they all eventually come out to the same place as long as you don't get caught up in the loops. Sometimes it's convenient when trying to lose paparazzi and sometimes hilarious when training assistants.

On the way, Walter filled me in on the vagaries of the job, as well as regaled me with stories of my new boss. One thing he cautioned me on was to make sure that I had money in hand before I made any financial commitments (like buying the ice). Walter and his friend, Gordon, were not too happy about using their own money for things and were pretty fed up with supporting Trygve's dream. One night after I knew them a bit, they told me the story of Trygve and Public Service to illustrate the lengths to which Trygve would go to secure funding for his dreams.

During the process of developing the area and building the facility, Public Service sent a survey team to mark out a location on the right-of-way for a new power pedestal. Some PS officials came out and carefully set their flags in the positions where the pad would be poured in the next few days. That night (or so the story went), Trygve went out and moved the flags ten feet to the side, off the right-of-way and onto his own property. He waited until they had poured the slab and set the transformer before he piped up and said that because they had built on his property and not on the right-of-way, they would owe him rent. Naturally, Public Service didn't take too kindly to this. (I always wondered if the surveyor ever got any flak for his "mistake.") But being the monopoly it is, PS dealt with it by saying that if Tryg was going to charge rent, he could pretty much suck on a pine tree for electricity. End of that story.

Another story that Walter told me was that the ice company he was using at the time was notorious for shorting the dry ice. I later found out that this was mostly due to how long the ice sits around before pickup. Dry ice is some pretty strange stuff, and I had to be careful of how I transported it. I had handled it in small quantities in college labs and later in dorm rooms with little thought on more than the chilling and explosive aspects of it. There are more subtle problems when you deal with large quantities. Posted on the door of the dry ice facility in Denver was a sign that read: "All personnel must wait a minimum of 30 minutes to enter warehouse after opening door for the first time in the morning." You have to be eighteen to even buy dry ice. I learned a lot about dry ice and a few other things those first couple of years.

THE EARLY YEARS AND THE DRY ICE WARS

The good Lord never gives you more than you can handle…unless you die of something.
—Guindon

The first time I made an official ice run, I almost killed myself. I had received the money and was going to go down to Denver to get the ice and meet up with Walter in Boulder before we would make the trip to Nederland. I was driving a Jeep Grand Wagoneer (sort of a large station wagon) at the time, and I was due to pick up four hundred pounds of ice. The ice runs were being made every two to three weeks with four hundred to six hundred pounds of dry ice because Trygve was afraid that something would happen if the facility was not checked on at least twice a month. It was in the early spring and it was a cold day. I had met the ice people, who were pretty nice (if only because I wasn't Trygve or Walter), and they loaded me up with a properly weighed load. I headed up the highway to Boulder with the radio on and the windows closed, blithely ignorant of the dangers of carbon dioxide in confined spaces. I had the heater on and the ice safely (so I thought) stored in the back, wrapped in insulation.

As I was driving the half hour or so to Boulder, I started to get a little sleepy and was yawning all over the place. I cracked the window and rather quickly felt more alert. I didn't really note anything out of the ordinary, but after rolling the window back up, I felt somewhat sleepy pretty quickly again. I made it to Walter's house, stumbled out of the car and immediately felt better. At that time, Walter made it clear to me that the sign on the warehouse door was not in jest. The carbon dioxide had been building up in the Wagoneer, and I was lucky that I didn't pass out. Being heavier than air and pretty much nonsupporting of life makes for some unusual properties and uses for dry ice. In fact, there are several sophisticated assassination techniques using dry ice that are efficient, quiet, deadly and virtually untraceable. In the lab, we would use it for critical point drying, a technique that sucks every last bit of moisture out of a specimen just using carbon dioxide. Nice stuff.

For the rest of that trip, and for every other trip in the Wagoneer, I always kept the tailgate window slightly down, as well as at least one other window (preferably the driver's) down at least an inch, no matter the weather or conditions. Eventually, I switched to a pickup truck, and the ventilation became moot.

When I started the ice runs, there was only one dry ice supplier in town. People might think that dry ice is available in multiple locations, but all of the dry ice in Colorado came through a single warehouse in Commerce City. One company, pretty much a monopoly, ruled the roost. It got whatever price it asked for; if you didn't pay, you didn't play. Trygve had worked out a commercial deal with the ice company and was getting a pretty good price, relatively speaking. And then, one day, a new outfit rode into town.

This new company, let's call them Company B, contacted me because its new general manager was the old company's (let's call it Company A) assistant general manager, and he had left to start the new company with some new people. It was getting its ice from a different source and could make me "such a deal." In truth, it offered me ice at half the price I had been paying. I had been working with Company A for almost two years, and Trygve and I had settled on a contract (after months of haggling) that paid me a flat amount each month for a certain amount of ice. The prospect of finding a new supplier on my own that could cut my costs almost in half—and *I* could still charge the same—was very appealing.

I had been in several heated discussions with Trygve by this time, trying for two years to deal with his financial acumen. He was always trying to get something for nothing (like the transformer pad) and was constantly asking me to do more and more for the same money. Essentially, he wanted to pay me for just doing the ice run while performing as a facilities manager, too. I was even making his mortgage payments for him. The money was wired directly into my account, and I would write checks to the mortgage company, as well as the ice company. The wires were not always on time. I could tell that Tryg was having trouble on the other end putting together the money to wire over. I had heard through the grapevine that Tryg's sister, who did not care for all of that cryonic nonsense, had come to Norway and convinced Aud to come and stay with her in Italy to get away from Tryg in Norway. Tryg was frantic to get her back, and that's when I found out about Aud's pension, which was what she and Tryg were using to support the facility. I figured that his sister was after the dough, too, and that it was just a family squabble. Eventually, Tryg got Aud back, and the money became more regular again.

One time, the payment was almost two weeks late. When I went into the mortgage office and asked to speak to the manager to explain, he filled me in on why there would be no late charges: "We live in absolute fear that Trygve will default on this loan," he said to me. "We so do not want to be stuck with a foreclosed monstrosity of a structure and a dead guy to boot!"

He said that they would bend over backward to ensure that Tryg made payments on time and that everything was financially stable—my first taste of the power of the Dead Guy. Eventually, Trygve was even able to convince the company to refinance and provide a better rate. He actually paid off the loan a few years ago and owns the place free and clear, or at least as free and clear as you can these days, considering taxes and the "Republic" of Boulder. But I digress.

So, when this new ice deal came along, I was ready to see if I could actually make a bit of profit off this job. Up to that time, I was barely making any. After expenses, gas, labor and all, I made about half what I should have been earning. This was an opportunity I couldn't pass up. So, I switched to Company B at half the price and inadvertently set off the "Denver Dry Ice Wars."

Company A did not take kindly to Company B taking away its customers. Company B was a tiny little upstart that should be squashed like a bug, according to the execs at the megacorporation. It did what any other big corporate giant in America would do, given the circumstances. It tried to drive B out of business by cutting its own prices to below Company B's prices, which was completely unsustainable. However, a megacorporation can afford to lose money for a little while in one small area if it means retaking the entire market by shutting down the competition. Deeper pockets are useful sometimes.

The only thing is that this turned into a real David v. Goliath story. When Company A cut its prices below cost and called all of Company B's customers, it really crossed the line. Company B took A to court and actually won the injunction for unfair business practices. Company A was pissed off, but there wasn't much it could do about it…or was there? Some might think that there was more to it, but I have always thought it was just divine providence, and maybe Bredo was laughing his ass off. About six months after the injunction, the nation's number one raw carbon dioxide producer bought out the only other producer in the country. Suddenly, it didn't really matter that there were two different dry ice entities in town—they both got all of their supplies from the same megacorporation.

Company A eventually bought the dry ice production equipment from Company B, and Company B moved its facility (now basically just shipping) to another location—at Company A. They operated together for several years, even though they were under court orders to stay away from each other. The order said that they couldn't harass each other. Technically, combining some of their services wasn't actually interfering in either's business and, in fact, turned out beneficial for everyone. Company B coexisted with Company A, saved facility expenses and got access to more distribution. Company A got a silent partner to defray expenses and its old employee back. I saved a couple bucks in gas and time, as Company A was ten miles closer to me than Company B. Everything else was exactly the same. Good ol' American business know-how.

So I finally got the dry ice thing settled down. Since Tryg only paid me a flat rate, getting ice at a cheaper price made the job profitable and interesting. Doing it in the summer was almost pleasant, in fact. The property had a great view of Barker Reservoir and the town of Nederland, and we'd bring up lunch, sit around and soak up the fresh mountain air for a spell before moving all of that ice. I usually went with one or two of my employees, and we all had fun going up into the mountains to deliver ice. During winter, it was a different story.

Carrying 400 to 500 pounds of dense dry ice in a truck that pulled up to the front door of the facility worked well. Having the place snowed in to one hundred yards away was not as good a prospect. These days, we carry more than 1,500 pounds of ice, and having to carry that much by hand through three feet of snow over the one hundred to two hundred yards, depending on how snowed in the place is, is really not a nice thing. In a blizzard, even. We eventually left a massive snowblower up at the property to clear the driveway for each trip with ice, and usually three guys can carry 500 pounds of ice in three trips. Solving that particular seasonal problem wasn't hard, especially for an ex–Transportation Corps officer like myself. We carried out

The Early Years and the Dry Ice Wars

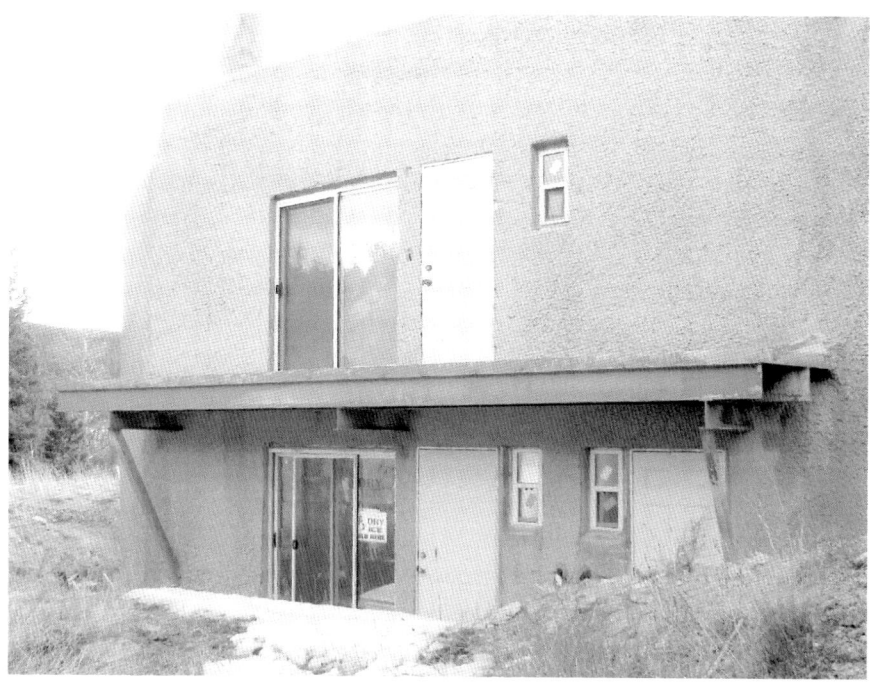

The bombproof, earthquake-proof, fireproof (everything but waterproof) Trygve-designed living space.

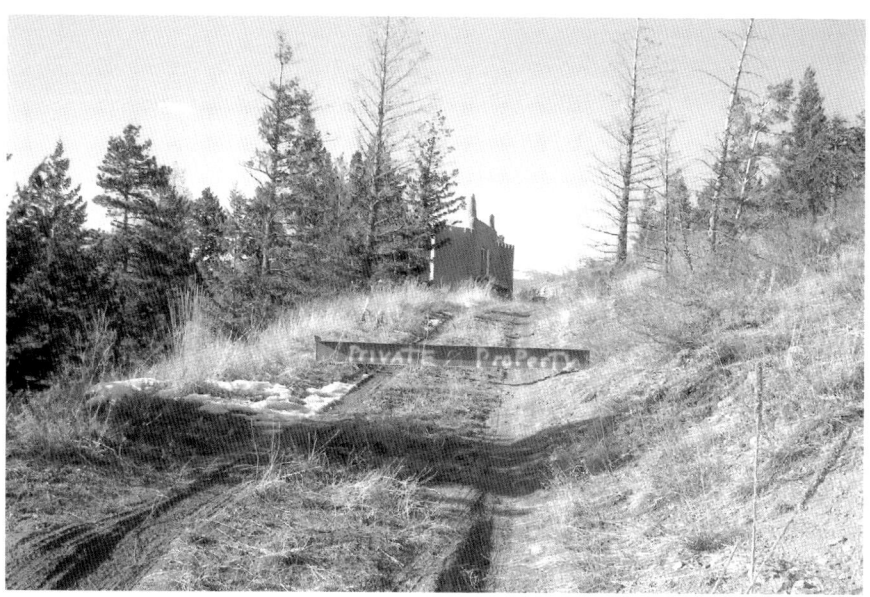

The institute driveway in summer.

the ice runs with military precision and dedication to the task. But sure as we solved one problem didn't another pop up.

The property was a bit strange: a sort of free-form cement main structure, which was Trygve's living quarters (now the IC Institute), a storage barn with a very bad roof and a couple of really cheap tin garden sheds with sliding panels for doors, side by side behind the main structure. There were a couple of old precast concrete tanks sitting at the base of the little cliff that formed the cutout for the property's structures. These were brought up to be septic tanks, but somehow they were broken on the trip—twice. Trygve had made some deal with the precast people to leave the broken tanks and had intended to make them into a hot tub and a cold plunge. Right next to the tanks were stacks of metal girders and specialty pieces of steel, made for the main structure and tunnels but never installed. Oh, did I mention that the whole place was supposed to be buried underground?

Trygve was a survivalist. He toured civil defense shelters, mines, caves and all kinds of seriously built and natural structures, looking at what ideas he could use to make his indestructible building. Fireproof, bombproof, earthquake-proof, cheap and easy to maintain—these were all important qualities to Trygve, and he wanted them to be included in his facility. Too bad that he didn't feel the same way about the cryonic storage chambers—the two tin sheds. I had pressed my crew into service and even my dear

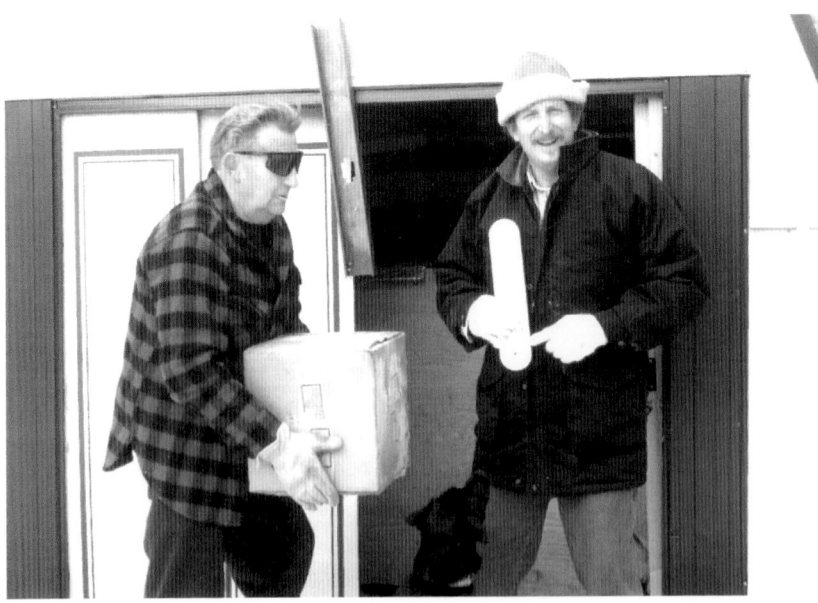

Bo and his father, Boyd, checking the temperature and loading boxes of dry ice.

The Early Years and the Dry Ice Wars

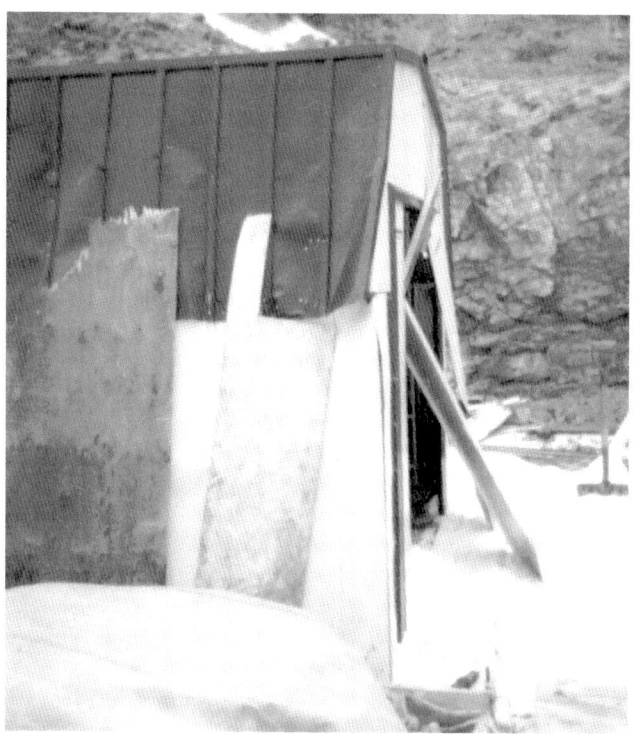

The original shed for Bredo, near the end of its existence.

ol' Da (he was a quarter Irish). Everybody thought that taking dry ice up and throwing it on a dead guy was hilarious. Pa got a big kick out of doing what was, in his estimation, crazy stuff. He was old school, but he had this streak of strangeness and a weird sense of humor that was probably the source of my own.

One time he was standing in line at a grocery store, and the lady in front of him forgot something. She asked my dad, standing with his family, to watch her four-year-old in the cart for just a second while she ran and got an item she forgot. My dad, the Crow Scout (opposite of an Eagle Scout), said, "Sure, no problem." After the mom left, my dad leaned over to the kid and said, "You know she's not coming back, right?" The kid's face turned white as a sheet, and he let out a squall that was heard all over the store. Everybody looked at him like he was some kind of child molester, and Pop was embarrassed as hell. We were all laughing like crazy. He had this way of making comments about things that were pretty off the wall sometimes. That Irish heritage. He's the one who made the comment about how the chains around the sarcophagus, used to lift it in and out, were really there to keep Grandpa in. I miss my old man's sense of humor.

Those winters were hellacious. Snow and wind every week it seemed. By December, all of the sheds were buried in several feet of snow, and the wind had taken its toll. The tin sheds were identical, sitting on a cement pad in this little cutout in the side of the mountain. The west shed was the cryonic storage building, and the east one was for storing everything else. Earlier that fall, the winds had completely destroyed the east shed, putting a piece of metal the size of a car hood up on top of the little twenty-foot cliff that overlooked the property. The nature of the cut allowed the fierce winds to roar in and swirl around, eventually forming a little whirlwind that was capable of picking up a fifty-pound piece of metal. The west shed was being beaten to pieces. Every time I'd find a piece missing, I'd screw some wood over the gaps. The sliding doors had stopped working, and I just screwed them into the main shed and unscrewed them every time I came to refill the ice. It was taking me more than twenty minutes just to get into the shed and another thirty minutes to realign all of the screw holes and screw the thing back together for another three weeks.

I didn't think that the shed would hold together much longer, and I was getting really tired of spending an extra hour just to deal with it. I complained to Walter, and he just shook his head and turned away. It seemed that there wasn't much he could do about it.

THE SHED THAT STARTED IT ROLLING

We've upped our standards, now up yours.
—Pat Paulson

One day in the spring of '95, Walter called me out of the blue and said that he had a friend who had an idea and that he wanted to run it past me. His buddy worked at a Denver rock radio station, and they were trying to figure out promotions for one of their new advertisers. The company was a local one, working on trying to get bigger (back in '95, Tuff Shed was not quite the nationwide company it is today; I like to think we had a little something to do with that), and the station had been doing some pretty imaginative promos. One was putting a DJ in a Tuff Shed up on a flagpole for a week—it got a bit of national attention. Another shed was put on top of a tall building in the dead of winter. Well, Walter had been telling his friend about our shed woes, and between the two of them over a late-night session, they came up with an interesting proposal.

A friend of Walter's, who was an advertising executive for Fox Radio, had talked Tuff Shed into donating a shed for Grandpa. He and Walter had worked out a promotional campaign that would run out over the radio for several weeks; one of the DJs would sort of take up our *cause célèbre*. Personally, I was stunned that someone actually wanted something to do with us, considering the reception we were used to in Ned and elsewhere. I had no inkling of what this was about to unleash.

We started out with a news story about me complaining about the conditions for "poor ol' Grandpa." We made a tiny notice in the back of

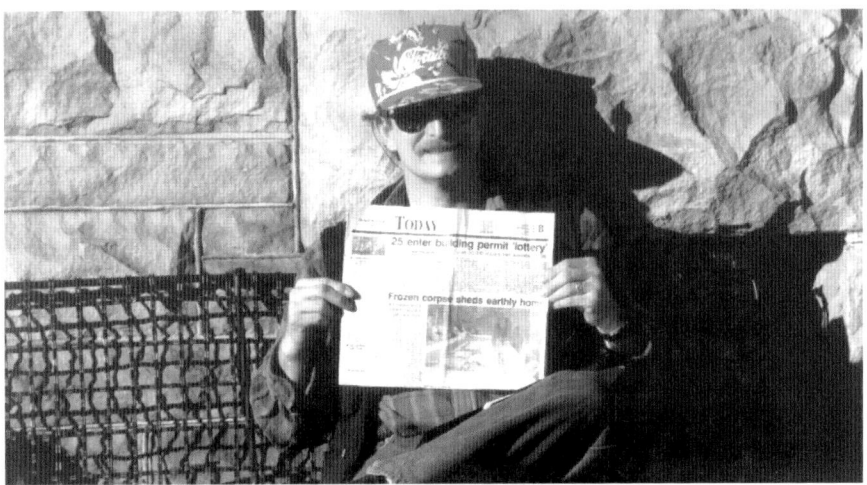

Bo holding up first newspaper headline about the "frozen corpse."

the local newspaper, but it was enough for the DJ to bring it out as a local interest story on his show and get the listeners involved. They talked about it off and on for more than a week, and then the DJ had the idea that maybe if the listeners and the DJ asked their advertiser, Tuff Shed, if there was any way that a new shed could be provided, there might be a chance of saving that poor dead grandpa. When he broke the news that Tuff Shed had agreed to donate a shed, he interviewed me on the air, and we talked about how difficult it was to run the operation with limited support and how grateful I was for the public's concern and help. In fact, we even had an opportunity for the public to get directly involved by calling for volunteers from the listening area to come up and help with the "conversion." Shades of Tom Sawyer! We even got headline newspaper coverage.

The day before the Tuff Shed was due to be delivered, about a dozen volunteers from all over the Fox Radio listening area showed up to help clean up the place and remove the remnants of the old tin shed from around Grandpa's cryonic chamber. We had drinks and snacks, the sun was out and we all had a great time, just hanging in the 'hood with Grandpa. Throughout the day's work, the one thing that everybody wanted to do was have a look into the chamber. So, after we knocked off for the day, we had a few beers and the crew gathered around while I removed the top to the chamber.

Back in those days, we didn't have no fancy-pants lid with newfangled things like hinges. No sirree Bob. We had seven layers of insulation and

The Shed that Started it Rolling

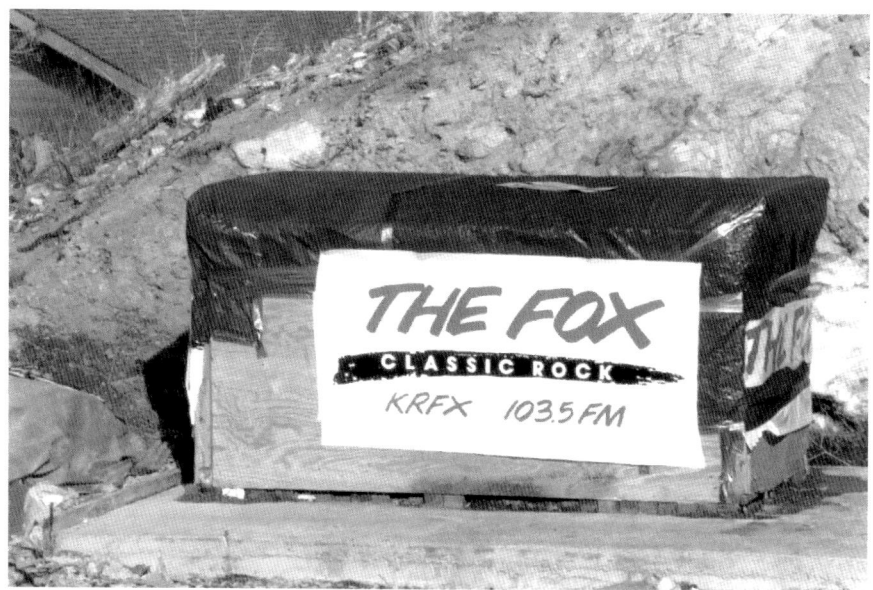

The cryonic chamber, with the old shed removed, sealed and labeled for the next day's erection of the new Tuff Shed.

plastic that had to be individually removed and (eventually) replaced. It was sort of like removing the bandages from a mummy. You unwrapped more and more and got closer and closer to what's underneath—but all in all, the job was a pain in the butt. It took about ten minutes to open it and fifteen to seal it back up. But once it was open and everyone could see the stainless steel sarcophagus, a bit of awe-struck silence held sway for just a minute. One of the volunteers, a black musician, looked in and said, "Damn! How you know he's really in there?" Looking back, I can't even begin to count the number of times I've been asked that question in the sixteen years I've been doing this. It is the second-most-asked question, posed by probably just about everyone who has ever looked into the cryonic chamber. Death just fascinates some people.

After everybody got a good look, we wrapped the chamber up in plastic, and everybody went home. Me and my crew, as well as my family, had all planned to come up the next day, bright and early, when the Tuff Shed boys would be there. They had planned to do the whole thing in one day, and so the sides were prefabricated, the walls were prepainted and the whole thing was stacked and transported up on a big flatbed truck. The promotions director of Tuff Shed was videotaping the entire process. Later, when we watched it again and sped it up a little, it was pretty wild watching this bunch of guys scurry all over the structure as it rose up like a growing thing out of flat nothing. After raising the sides and power-nailing the frame to the cement, they put on the roof pieces and doors and started shingling it. Even with a power-nailer, the shingling took almost as much time as the rest of the job. But

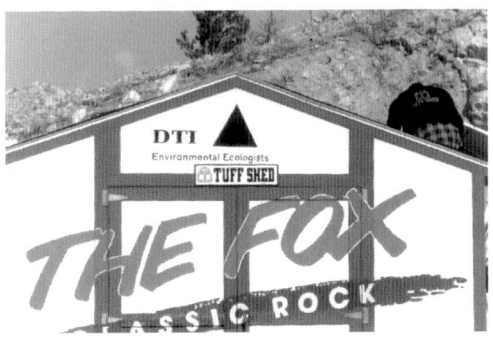

A Tuff Shed worker finishing the roof of the brand-new shed.

when they were done, a magnificent new Tuff Shed—with a custom, hand-painted exterior—stood in all its splendor. The shed even had a solar panel and a light. That was more than could be said for the main building.

Oh, did I mention that every local TV news channel had a mobile rig up there for the big event? The campaign was thorough and well thought out. Practically every person with a TV in the Greater Denver area knew that Tuff Shed had donated one of its sheds to Grandpa because it was the toughest shed on the market and was critical to our needs. Everybody was interviewed, and even my family got in the video as the Tuff Shed boys handed over the keys and we inspected the result. Nice!

As nice as it was, however, there were a couple of flaws that would soon be pointed out by the inimitable County of Boulder government. Since I was the general contractor for this job, the Tuff Shed boys came, built and split. I was left to schedule the inspection and finish up the little details. When the inspector inspected, the shed failed to have hurricane clips and anchor bolts. "Toenails and power nails don't cut it in Boulder County," he said. So I installed the clips and bolts and brought it up to Boulder County standards. If you look at the Boulder building code map of wind design, you'll see a tiny circle around the Nederland area. Things are more stringent when it comes to designing windproof structures, and after what had happened to the auxiliary tin shed, I was inclined to agree with them. The other flaw was a bit more esoteric.

Apparently, due to the nature of the custom paint job—basically a giant radio station logo on each side of the shed—it was considered a "sign," and as such…we had no sign permit. After wrangling with Boulder County officials over this (much like wrestling a pig, you get nowhere and the pig

The Shed that Started it Rolling

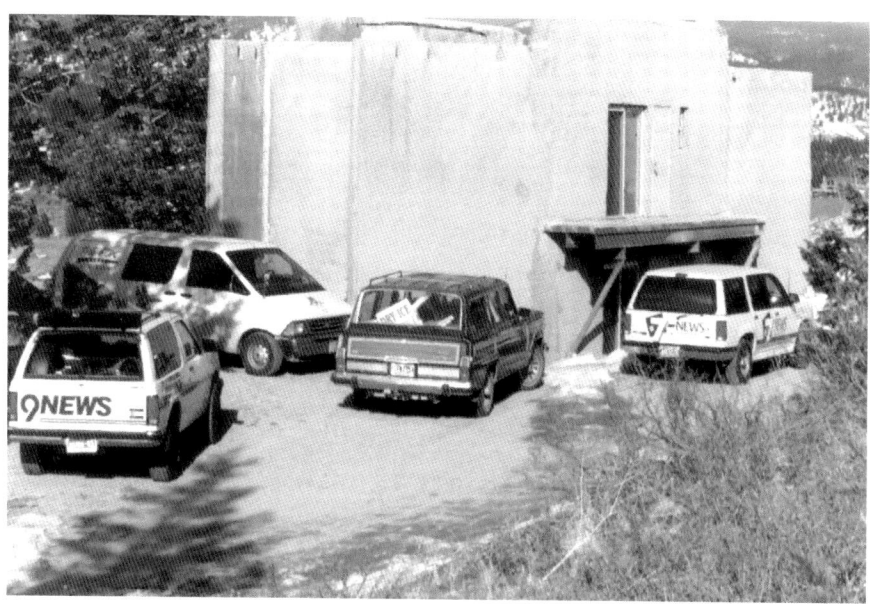

The media frenzy whipped up for the new Tuff Shed for Grandpa.

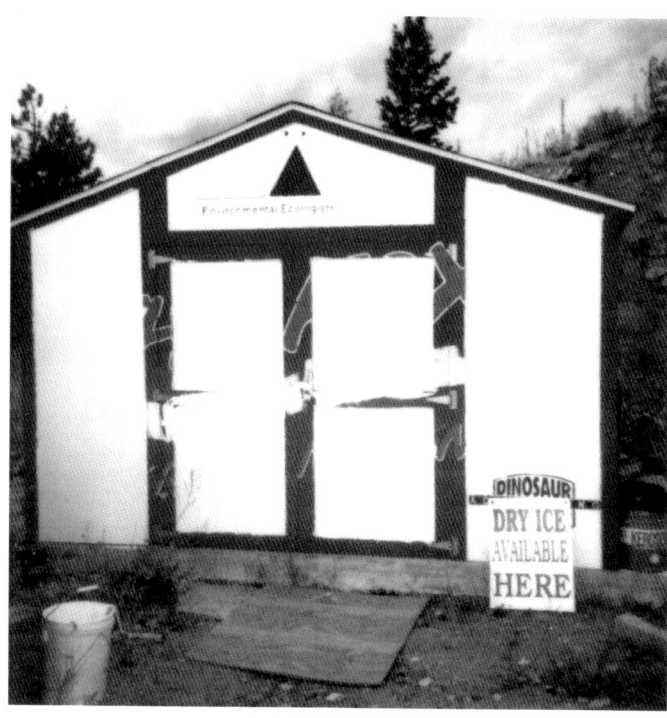

The new shed, with the nonconforming sign portion painted over.

seems to enjoy it), I finally got them to accept me painting most of each of the three sides that were actually visible "off the property" (as per ordinance language). I painted the panels but not the trim, so there was a little bit of the logo visible, but it was no longer legible. I left the back wall as it was, because no one can see this wall from anywhere but right next to it, as it faces a twenty-foot cliff face.

For many years, the favorite video at Tuff Shed's trade shows was the sped-up video of the shed's construction. We even made it into one of its national commercials, though you wouldn't really know what it was. If you ever see a Tuff Shed commercial in which the Tuff Shed flatbed truck is driving away from you, down a mountain dirt road, and the guys inside stick their arms out and wave goodbye, that was the crew that built Grandpa's shed as they drove away that afternoon. I hear the company still uses that clip in some of its commercials.

It really was after this that things started to change a bit for the better. Having a corporate sponsor, so to speak, put us up there with a little dash of credibility. We were looking good for the first time since I had started this crazy job. The word was getting around that there was this really weird thing up in (of all places) Nederland—sort of a local phenom. All of those people who complained way back when didn't seem to care as much now that they had a somewhat different perspective. Soon, word reached the infamous Beeck sisters…and things changed for good.

MEDIA COVERAGE SPREADS THE WORD

In the long run, we are all dead.
—John Maynard Keynes

Once every couple of years, some new person from one of the TV stations would call and want to do a ride along or interview or something for a human interest story. I would usually meet the reporter and cameraman at the dry ice place (whichever one it happened to be at the time), and they would shoot some footage of me loading the ice and the steam coming off the ice in the back of a car full of ice—all the fun things that one does when one moves a potentially deadly substance. Sometimes the reporter would ride along with me, and sometimes they would meet me up in Nederland. It would usually show up on the evening news, and I would get a big kick out of seeing myself and would always try to tell my friends to keep their eyes open that day as we made the six o'clock news again. Once the Tuff Shed came along, and we looked like a real bona fide cryonic storage facility and not just someone's garden shed, we actually started to look good on the nightly news.

I knew that we made the "big time" when I got a call from the *National Enquirer*. Like the "men in black" said, you can get a lot of knowledge out of that rag. The *Enquirer* reporter talked to me on the way up and said that we needed an angle. I asked him what kind of an angle, and he said, "A hook, you know, something to get the readers' attention." Just about that time, we were passing the liquor store in Ned, and he looked over and said, "That's it!" He asked me to pull over, and he ran inside and came out with a bottle wrapped in paper. On the way up to the shed, he pulled out a bottle of Old Grandad and said that we had to do a toast. If you were to see the article (I have a couple copies), you'd see the photo of the first-ever toast with Old Grandad over dry ice to Grandpa's picture. That was also when we invented the Frozen Dead Guy, a drink made quite popular later on at the festivals and tours. Oh, and just for the *Enquirer*, I wore my black "Kill 'em all…Let God sort 'em out" T-shirt. It's a classic photo.

People in Nederland started to know who I was. I would stop at the same doughnut shop every time I came up for an ice run, and the owner who baked his own goods got to know me pretty well. I was pretty leery of the town still, since they were supposedly all freaked out over having this dead body in the vicinity. But somehow the word was getting around—first the local news channels and then the occasional odd show. *Strange Universe* was one. It had gotten a whiff of the unusual and sent a reporter to check it out. Once in a while, you'll see the show on late-night TV. Sometimes, though, the things that happened would be pretty cool, like the time I got to meet A. Whitney Brown.

I had gotten a call from a producer from Comedy Central who said that it had a show that was doing news, especially offbeat news, and wondered if I'd like to be on *The Daily Show*. Now, at that time, *The Daily Show* was hosted by Craig Kilborn and not Jon Stewart. He was more mock news and humorous commentary on the news than Stewart's political satire. Well, he sent out one of the show's roving reporters, who did features every week, and it turned out to be A. Whitney Brown. I had always liked him when he was on *Saturday Night Live*, with his dry sense of humor and delivery. So, even though I was a little concerned about being made a laughingstock on Comedy Central, I agreed to do an interview with Brown. The producer had heard about the psychic things we did (more about that later) and wanted to locate a couple of local psychics to go along with Brown. I gave her the names of a few local psychic networks, and she said that she'd check them out.

The day of the ice run dawned, and the entourage showed up: a cameraman, a sound man, a producer, two psychics and "the talent." Along with myself and my assistant, we filled up three vehicles. We got up there, and it was a perfect day, if just a bit windy. Gave the sound man a fit. But, all in all, it went pretty well. The so-called psychics, however, were not so hot. They said that they sensed Grandpa being tired of all the hoopla and that he just wanted to be at rest. I think they had an agenda and wanted to get it on national TV. "The poor spirit should be left alone and put to rest." How wrong they were. A. Whitney was in rare form, and the segment turned out pretty funny, especially the "gay repartee" between him and Kilborn.

Globo International, a news magazine–format TV show out of Brazil, also brought up a psychic. That one was much more believable. When you deal with dead guys, the psychics crawl out of the woodwork. This brings me to a small but relevant point of trivia. Up to this time, everybody had been talking about a "frozen corpse" or, as A. Whitney put it, "a frozen corpsicle" or perhaps "frozen Grandpa." My then five-year-old son, Morgan, was doing speech therapy for a very unusual speech impediment that was just about gone. He was very happy to be reading and sounding just like everybody else, and he read out loud from the paper about frozen Grandpa and his dad. He just thought it was so cool. He and I talked about just what it was sometimes at night before bed. I always made it a point to be there at bedtime if I could. It was my favorite time of the day to spend with the kids. With Morgan, I was the "Big Guy" and he was the "Little Guy." We'd play a little game about how many superlatives we could add to stretch out the goodnights, describing each "guy." When Morgan and I talked about Grandpa Bredo, we just naturally started calling him the frozen dead guy, and it just kind of slipped in and stuck. I remember the Globo people trying to translate "frozen dead guy" into Portuguese. Came out more like "congealed expired dude."

The media event that sort of blew it all open, though, was a combination of two things at the right time and the right place. First, in the fall of 2000, I had been contacted by a young Boulder filmmaker by the name of Robin Beeck, who was interested in making a film about Grandpa Bredo and the Tuff Shed. Robin had made two other documentaries before this, and I had actually seen one of them. I had been involved with the CU Film Studies Department for many years. I used to do repair work on the department chairman's house and hang out with him by his pool up in the really nice part of old Boulder. One day, after I had fixed a particularly difficult electrical problem, we got to talking about documentaries, and he eventually suggested that I come to an evening showing of this documentary about Alaska by one of his students. He said that it was pretty well done and won an award. I ended up being in town that evening and went and saw it. It was a remarkable documentary of one man's struggle and how he copes with losing the Iditarod. I was impressed. So, when I got this call from Robin asking me if I would mind if she made this documentary about Grandpa, I was flattered and agreed. Of course, the fact that she was quite easy on the eyes and had several sisters didn't hurt, either. My assistants were pretty excited when they heard that they might get into the movies with a bunch of female film fanatics. Little did we know that we were just pawns in a much bigger game.

Robin was sweet and talented. She had made a second documentary since I had seen her first. This one was about the city of Boulder. It was well received, too. She had a simple, down-to-earth way of telling a story with her voice and camera. In fact, she was so good that she was awarded a $10,000 grant from director Michael Moore to do her next documentary—about the frozen dead guy. She and I worked for hours together thinking about shots and going up to the shed to shoot scenes. We even went up in a blizzard to get shots with snow in them. We used my Wagoneer as a mobile camera platform a few times, too—the camera sat on the back, and we slowly backed up to the shed as the doors opened. I liked what she had done with the other documentaries, and I felt that this one would be good, too. However, the second media event was timed to hit right at that creative moment when artists are receptive, and it was such a bright one that it kind of temporarily blinded some people.

Extra!, the flashy, nationally syndicated news magazine–format TV show, had called up and wanted to do a show on the Beecks and the frozen dead guy. I had no idea that this had all been prearranged as a jumping-off point for publicizing Robin's (soon to be "the Beeck sisters") yet-unfinished documentary *Grandpa's in the Tuff Shed*. I was used to having film crews up at the shed, but several times, Trygve had complained about crews stealing his stuff and getting free pictures and souvenirs. I had strict rules about always being present whenever anyone was on the property. When Robin and I started out, it was just she and I. It was great, doing artistic shots and doing certain shots over and over to get it just like she wanted it. I felt like we were getting the story out in a really interesting way. Her father came up a couple times just to lend support. It was a nice family-supported project.

It was about this time that her sisters, having Moore's grant firmly in mind, decided that their dear little sister was going to make them a whole lot more money than they could running a cleaning service or dealing with failed businesses and relationships. So they decided to move in and help manage her career. The first move was for the *Extra!* interview, with all three girls pushing the film they had hoped to submit to the International Film Festival. I had told the girls that I would meet them at a certain time up at the shed and had arranged with the *Extra!* producers to meet them at my favorite doughnut shop. When I got to the doughnut shop, nobody was there. It turned out that the Beeck sisters had come by an hour earlier because they apparently had called ahead for the crew to come up an hour earlier and then took them all up to the shed by themselves.

By the time I got to the shed myself, I was not in a very good mood. When I saw the girls with the camera crew and saw that they had been running all around, moving things without me being there, as my job required, I kind of lost it on their asses. I chewed them out for a minute or two right in front of the big-time producer from New York whom the girls were trying so hard to impress. To this day, Shelly Beeck looks daggers at me every time she sees me. She never forgave me for embarrassing her in front of that producer.

After that session, I didn't see much of the girls. When I got the first cut of *Grandpa's in the Tuff Shed*, I couldn't believe what I saw. Not a single mention of me in any of the credits. None of the difficult footage from the snowstorm and the mobile platform was in the cut. The soundtrack was unlike either of the other documentaries that Robin had done. The music was incidental in those but driving and compelling in this one—funny, just like the *Extra!* soundtrack. I was identified as an "ice delivery person," and that was the only mention of my name, or my company's name, anywhere in the film. Hell hath no fury as a woman embarrassed in a prestige-conscious industry, especially when she's the film editor. It was funny, too: about 90 percent of the credits were all Beecks. Seemed like every Beeck in the family, from grandpa on down to all the grandkids, had a credit for something. But no mention of me or my company, Delta Tech, or anything. Months later, after stewing about it all for a while, I noticed that the final copy released for the film festival had some slightly different credits than the original one, which I still have in my archives. A study in angry women, I suppose.

As for a newer version, *Grandpa's Still in the Tuff Shed*, it's a study in crass commercialism. Take a winning film, add a bunch of unrelated stuff to it and then sell it again. This is especially true when you manufacture a plotline. Bredo's ghost has never been seen in Colorado, because he had very little to do with the area when he was alive. Most ghosts have attachments to where they haunt. Hooking several of the town's more colorful people into pushing this fake story about ghosts doesn't make for a better movie in my estimation.

But that's what happens when the marketing and sales people take over from the artistic types. It loses its soul.

The original *Grandpa's in the Tuff Shed* went over pretty well. The one music track that was better than the rest was Chip and the Chowderheads singing "Grandpa's in the Tuff Shed, chillin' to the bone." (I remember they played it several times at the first Blue Ball.) It had a great tag line, but it got old rather quickly. *Extra!* promoted the film and it won awards. It was a hit locally, and it had national coverage—international coverage even. Not much, but it really was just that kind of a story. All in all, it was the collision of two media events that really put Grandpa on the map, so to speak. Because of this, one day much later, the members of the Nederland Chamber of Commerce sat around and had a few drinks and came up with an idea.

MOMENTUM INCREASES WITH THE FDGD

The best audience is intelligent, well educated, and a little drunk.
–Alben W. Barkley

The members of the Nederland Chamber of Commerce were sitting around one winter day discussing the Spring Fling that they tended to have every year to relieve the locals' cabin fever. They needed a theme, and one of them brought up Mike the Headless Chicken of Fruita, Colorado—home to a festival celebrating its most famous resident, Mike. Back in the 1950s, a freak head-lopping left Mike with most of his faculties intact. He could walk and run but had a little bit of a hard time eating with basically no head and just a pie hole. But he lived eighteen months, and it's documented. Pictures and everything. These days, the Mike the Headless Chicken Festival is quite a local hit and more than a little colorful. So someone from the chamber brought up the bright idea of celebrating Nederland's weirdest resident with a Frozen Dead Guy Days Festival. Somehow this idea sounded better after a couple of draughts at the Pioneer Inn, so eventually the chamber representative contacted me to run it by me and see what I thought.

Theresa Warren was an activist in Nederland. She was a business owner and had recently taken over the chair position on the Nederland Chamber of Commerce. She was really hoping for something to lift the economy of Nederland and had been working her tail off to make it happen. She had a list of interesting-sounding events, like a Coffin Race and a Polar Plunge. She said that the race would be open to the public, with rewards going to

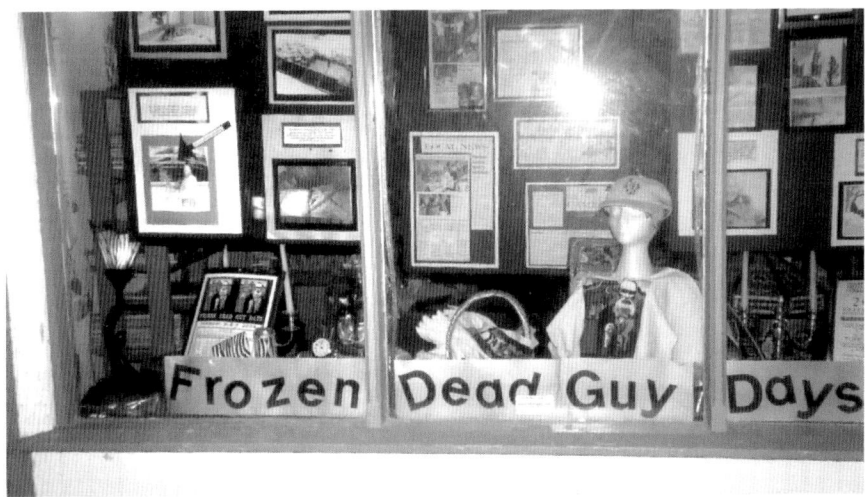

The "History of the Frozen Dead Guy" window display at Off Her Rocker.

imagination as much as race ability. Something like the Kinetics Race meets pallbearers with a bobsled. I thought it had potential.

I was thinking that it would be fun to have people up to the shed, so we talked about having tours. The Polar Plunge event was in tribute to Trygve as much as the frozen dead guy. Trygve was deeply into the life extension thing, and ice plunges were part of his regimen. In fact, Trygve held the Guinness world record for sitting in an ice bath for more than an hour. Of course, his head and arms, with hands clasped behind his head, weren't in the water, but still…pretty impressive. So eventually I contacted Trygve, told him about the pending festival and asked if he would consent to having tours up at the property. Since it furthered Trygve's constant quest for international fame, he readily agreed, as long as I would be present at all times.

Theresa and I and the other chamber members put our heads together and worked out a feasible plan for a festival. Her husband, Brent, was a pretty good artist but was making a living doing other things. She was able to get him to do the original artwork for a pittance (which was all the chamber could afford), and thus the iconic image of an old bearded guy with icicles came into being, along with the Red Ball. She also did a big display of all of the media articles and photographs in the front window of her shop on Main Street, Off Her Rocker.

So the first festival was pretty much on a shoestring. No one knew for sure if it would even work. Maybe folks would be turned off by such a macabre concept for a party. But if it was good enough for Oingo Boingo, then let's go ahead and "Party with a Dead Man." That song pretty much gets played somewhere during the festival every year—sort of the unofficial theme song of the Frozen Dead Guy Days. I wonder if Danny Elfman would like to come and sing his song at the festival some day? Probably not, as I hear that he doesn't do live stuff anymore because his ears were pretty blown out by all of that high-intensity stuff with the Mystic Knights of Oingo Boingo, and he's afraid he'll go deaf. Well, he does make a living off being able to hear, I suppose. But wasn't Beethoven deaf? At any rate, music was always intended to be part of the festival. And films, too.

The Beeck sisters' film was one of the festival's main attractions, being all tied up with Michael Moore and everything. This FDGD was actually the impetus for them to start the Boulder International Film Festival (BIFF). *Grandpa's in the Tuff Shed* played to a full house all weekend. They got Chip and the Chowderheads to play at the ball. Sponsors were sparse but obvious. Tuff Shed was a big one. The company got a lot of mileage out of Grandpa over the years. But we got a Tuff Shed. We're about even. Eldora was a surprise sponsor. Over the years, members of that company turned out to be really into the whole thing and even trucked snow some years from the slopes to the racecourse. The chamber of commerce was a sponsor, of course, and the Town of Nederland itself—and that was it. Four sponsors. The town was donating space and venues, and Eldora and Tuff Shed were

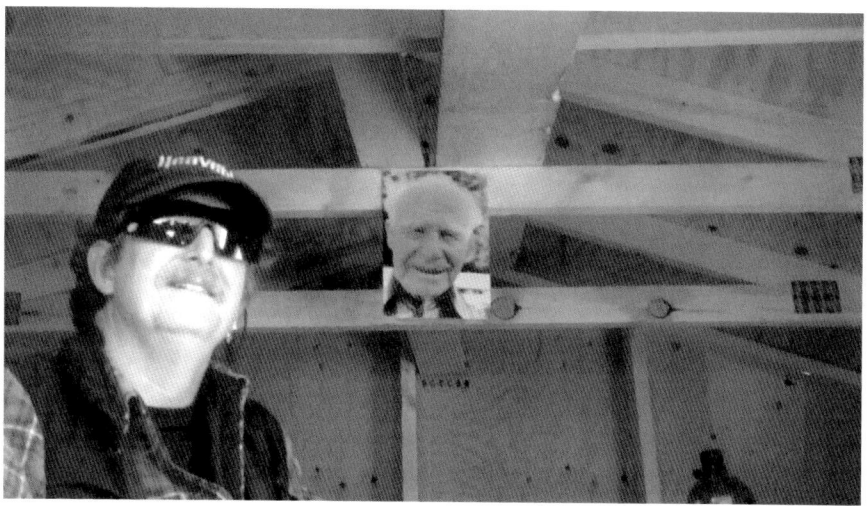

Bo posing with Bredo for the promo shots on the first tour.

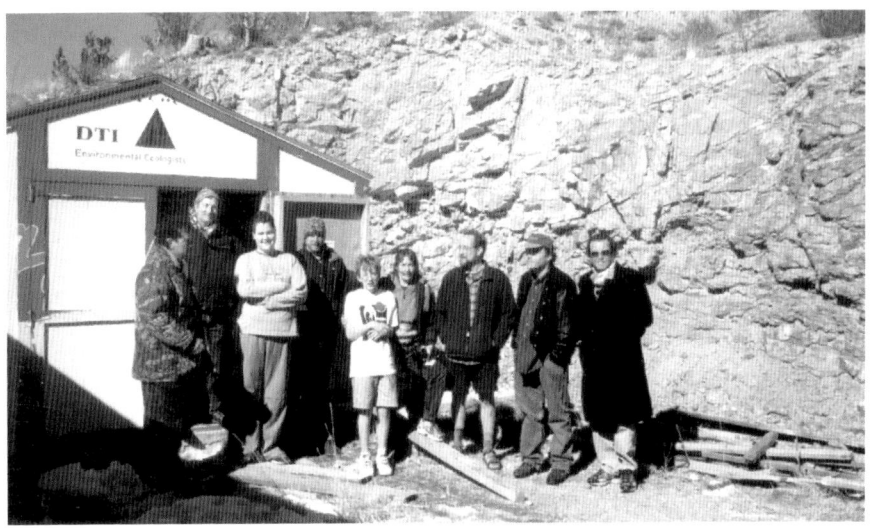

The first tour group.

the financial backers. The chamber beat and flogged their volunteers to do the work of three times as many people as they had. Debbie, Hughs, Serene and everyone else did whatever was necessary to make this thing fly, and somehow it all came together.

The first year it was Saturday and Sunday only. It opened with the pancake breakfast and went right into the parade. I had tours on both days, but the first official tour of the cryonic facility was for half media. Great for publicity but bad for the pocketbook having to comp so many tickets. Later on, we had all paying customers, even a teenage kid in shorts. Crazy kid. There were a couple dozen Coffin Race entries, and everyone knew all about the Kinetics Sculpture and Race event in Boulder, where the costumes were as important as actually winning the race. As many points for decorations as ability made sure that people would go for goofy if they couldn't do power. They didn't disappoint. I got to be in the parade, too, that time. Grandpa's Secret Other Ball was on Saturday night and turned into one of the biggest events in the ensuing years. All in all, it turned out a lot better than anyone thought it would. But what it really did was set the stage for 2003.

In 2003, everyone was hyped up about the festival. Brent's theme poster was the bearded Grandpa figure holding an ice cream cone, standing in front of the Nederland Town Hall (which is an extremely rustic-looking wooden cabin), with the Red Ball sun sinking into the mountains. I did radio interviews with people all over the world in the weeks leading up to the big weekend. Did a few in the good ol' United States, too. There was lots of interest in the Midwest for some reason, probably the proximity to Colorado and the possibility that they just might even get to go there. The Beeck sisters went and made a "new" movie called *Grandpa's Still in the Tuff Shed* and filled it up with all sorts of fluff and hype for Nederland—ghosts, indeed—but it did bring out several other filmmakers, and they were actually able to hold the first (now annual) Frozen and Dead Film Festival at the Backdoor Theater. Their comment about this making Nederland like "Mayberry in the Twilight Zone" was a good one.

The entries were all on the theme of dead and frozen. John Barnard brought his *Cemetery Love Story*, all about digging up parts of a dead guy. Eric Patrick's *Ablution*, which played to much critical acclaim in Europe and Australia, was another highlight. Then there was *If Spielberg Made a Snuff Film* and *Daypass*, both of which came from New York City film fests with wins and honorable mentions. Even Trygve got on board with the film fest thing and submitted a video of his activity in Norway. We got to watch him prepare for his ice bathing and then watched as he went out in the snow and ice and chopped down a tree to get to the place where he wanted to chop out the ice. Not the greenest actions I've ever seen, but then it's Norway, and I believe they have no real shortage of trees. There was also a hilarious segment with Tryg being interviewed on a Norwegian show about life in the United States. Last, but certainly not least, I submitted a short documentary consisting of video clips from all of the people who had done shows on us: *National Geographic*, *Extra!*, *Comedy Central*, *Ripley's Believe It or Not!*, *Strange Planet*, Globo International and more. I narrated it during the showing, and it was well received; everyone thought that it was a fascinating history of the often bizarre case of the frozen dead guy.

We also had our first celebrity visitor, Bill Geist. Bill did a show called *The Sunday Morning* show on national TV. His people had contacted us about him attending for a bit on Friday or Saturday, and we had talked them into helping to emcee the Grandpa Look-alike Contest on Saturday afternoon (he actually entered himself in the finals that night and took honorable mention) and then talked him into being the presenter at the Frozen and Dead Film Fest on Sunday. Basically, he intended to stay for a few hours and ended up spending the entire weekend at the festival. I think it actually gave him the idea for his book, *Way Off the Road*. Naturally, we ended up being one of the featured communities (page 42), being so in tune with the title and all.

Colorado's Iceman

With Bill Geist as a celebrity draw, the video fest coordinator (one of the many hats that Theresa wore) went all out Hollywood-style. We had a searchlight, tuxedos, red carpets, champagne and the first-ever world premiere of a film in Nederland. It's amazing what a little PR can do for a tiny event. The rest of the town was starting to warm up to Grandpa and the whole dead guy thing. The town's ice cream parlor made a special blend and called it Cryogenic Crunch. The B&F Market ran its weekly advertisements in the local paper adorned with icicles and touting such things as "Headless Shrimp" and "Whole Dead Rotisserie Chicken" and, of course, Tombstone Pizza. That local paper, the *Mountain Ear*, had a reporter, Barbara Lawlor, who had been around since the beginning and was always there to take pictures and write stories about all of the strange things inspired by the frozen dead guy. She had as much as anyone to do with promoting the concept.

One of the most interesting events added to this year's festival (at least from my perspective) was the Midnight Champagne Tour. Spawned in the somewhat inebriated aftermath of the first festival tours and Grandpa's Ball, I decided to take advantage of the fact that the more intoxicated folks got, the more everybody wanted to go and see Grandpa. Worked for me. I couldn't figure out how to charge, though, since this was strictly a bootleg operation with no official sanction. In the end, I took my cue from Robin Hood. I charged you whatever you had, tempered with whether I really wanted you along or not. Real drunks and annoying people got charged fifty bucks, regular folks paid whatever they had. Over the years I've been paid everything from a fifth of Old Grand-Dad Special Label to a can of Monster energy drink. Pretty girls can often come along for just a kiss, depending on whether my wife is around or not. The key thing for going on the Midnight Champagne Tour is finding me that night at the ball. Sort of like the Zulu parade in New Orleans during Mardi Gras. You have to know someone to find out where the parade route goes. If you don't know me, you have to know someone who knows me to find me and get included on the tour. When you find me, and I accept your bribe, I tell you the exact time and place we'll meet to head out to the shed later that night. Over the years, we have had some epic Midnight Champagne Tours.

The first inaugural Midnight Champagne Tour had been arranged for the owner and the general manager of Tuff Shed and their respective ladies. I got a very cool coat from the Tuff Shed guys, complete with the Tuff Shed logo on the back and my name embroidered on the front. I was told that I was the only person at that time who had that jacket and didn't

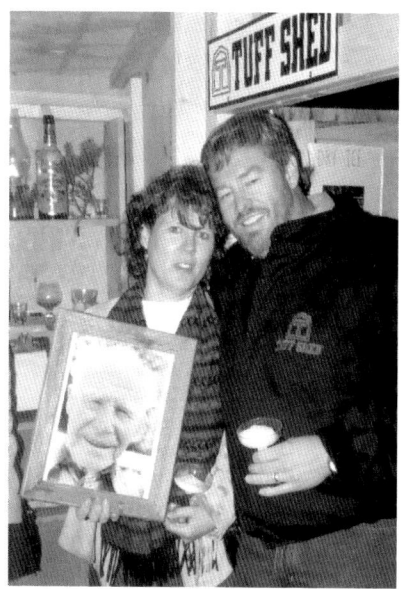

The owner of Tuff Shed and his lady at the first inaugural Midnight Champagne Tour.

work for Tuff Shed. It turned out to be the warmest, lightest coat I've ever had, and I usually wear it during every festival. While I was waiting at the ball for my party to gather, a couple of high rollers from New York City who had stumbled upon the festival while driving around the mountains asked if they could come, too. They had a bottle of really good champagne to offer, and thus the Midnight Champagne Tour was born out of serendipity. Events with champagne later that night would set the name as a memorial for every tour since.

Always looking for angles and promos as we started out the tour, I thought it would be a cool idea to put the champagne on dry ice in the cooler on the way up to the shed, to cool it down faster and also have the tie-in with Grandpa and his dry ice. It only takes about ten minutes to drive from the center of town to the facility. But by the time we got up there, unloaded everybody, opened the shed and were ready to have a toast to Grandpa, the champagne had a good half hour in the cooler with the dry ice.

When something is cooled quickly, at a very low temperature, some interesting things can happen. While it tends to preserve tissues and (hopefully) bodies, it tends to supercool liquids with antifreeze in them—like the champagne with its intrinsic alcohol. "Supercooling" is a term used to describe the phenomenon of a liquid cooling to below its freezing point yet remaining liquid. Eventually, it does freeze and, if contained in small spaces, can explosively be released through the destruction of the containment vessel, the way sodas and beer explode in your freezer. Fortunately for us that night, champagne bottles are thicker than regular wine bottles and are meant to withstand considerable pressure. Even so, when we finally popped the cork on the bottle, it literally exploded with a fountain of partially frozen champagne spewing all over the cryonic chamber and all over Bredo's sarcophagus. The place stunk like a frat party aftermath for months. The cork, however, had a mind of its own.

For any of you old enough to remember a cartoon by the name of "Ricochet Rabbit," you will have some idea of the cork's wild flight. *Ping… ping…ping, ping, PING!* It hit several times in the small confines of the Tuff Shed, but the last ping was off a portrait of Bredo that hangs above the cryonic chamber and is in a particularly solid wood frame that weighs several pounds. It was at that time held up with just one nail in the back like a regular picture (now it is secured with several three-inch screws and checked periodically for looseness). The cork knocked the picture off the nail, and it fell right into the hand of the guy who was responsible for building the shed, Dan Meinerz, general manager of Tuff Shed. Dan gave a little yelp but caught the picture and said that it was okay and to go on with the toast. I poured what was left of the champagne in the bottle into glasses, and as I was passing them out to everyone, I looked down at Dan's hand. It was pretty much covered in blood, bleeding like a stuck hog and dripping all over the floor of the shed. The corner of the picture had put a gash in his hand and nicked a vein to boot—not gushing bright-red blood but rather lots of the oozing, dark-red, clotting kind. We put some regular ice and a compress on it, but it dripped for quite a long time.

We didn't have much in the way of equipment to clean and dress the wound, so we wrapped it up and planned to take care of it when we got back to town. Dan helped put things back together inside the shed, and there are still bloodstains to be seen on the floor and some of the insulation on the chamber. It wasn't until the next month's ice run that I found the cork, wedged into the far corner of the cryonic chamber, and left it there for posterity. Every cork has a story, I guess. This one is all about how a dead guy jumped off the wall and "bit" the hand that made his house. Maybe Bredo was making a statement. Maybe he just got drunk with that shot of champagne and fell into the guy accidentally. Who's to say? There were a lot of traditions and tales that started in the second annual Frozen Dead Guy Days that continue to this day. Time will tell how long they persist.

In 2004, the festival got off to an unusual start when a rumor of Trygve's death made the rounds, and people were all shook up, wondering what could possibly have happened. I hadn't heard from Tryg in several months leading up to the festival, even though I had sent several e-mails. Due to the fact that we only got paid for doing the ice runs once a month, and everything else we did was gratis, I was not one to spend money on phone calls to Norway. I pretty much communicated with Trygve exclusively by e-mails, at least from my end. Unfortunately, Tryg had this rather annoying habit of calling first thing in the morning (for him), which was the middle of the night for me. And he had my home number, so I couldn't really get away from him that way, either. He would call two or three times a day sometimes, mostly to make sure that things were okay and to get a report on every little detail of what happened.

One time, he even had me take a special phone up to the property during an ice run and call him to describe to him the contents of every box stored in the storage sheds and upstairs at the main structure. Somewhere around four to five hundred boxes. After about fifty boxes, I told him that this was the most ridiculous thing I had ever done and that if he wanted me to do it he was going to have to pay me a whole lot more than the nothing he was paying me at that time, because the ice run was done. He finally agreed with me that it was a waste of his money to do such a thing, but every so often he would ask about one of those fifty boxes we did catalogue. People with OCD are fun to work with but not so fun to work for.

His money was shipped automatically with a bank-to-bank transfer, and as long as the money came, I was doing the job and didn't have to talk to him. Over the years, there were many periods of several months or more when I wouldn't hear from Trygve and would send him e-mails and get no responses. He once told me that he only checked his e-mail four to five times per year. Considering the enormousness of Trygve's Meta Portal, his website for everything, one would think that he spent hours every day adding links and updating info. But when one checks out the site, one notices that it is stale and has many broken links. So it really wasn't that unusual to not have heard from Tryg for a couple months, although he usually had quite an interest in the festival, and it was a bit odd that he hadn't responded to some questions of mine about the tours.

That Friday, when I got to Ned, several people came up to me and asked me if I had heard about Trygve. I had no idea what they were talking about. That's when I heard about the rumor going around that Trygve had died and that the fate of the frozen dead guy was suddenly up for consideration. With the festival starting to catch on, everyone was worried that this would put the kibosh on things and spell the doom of both Bredo and the festival. Eventually, someone called Tryg and found out that his computer had broken down and that he had been on vacation in the fjords for the last month, so everyone was able to breathe a little easier. It did raise speculation, though, about what would happen if something happened to Tryg—or to Aud, for that matter, as she is really the one who finances this.

As far as I know, it's her substantial pension that keeps the money flowing to the United States every month. If the money stopped, would there be anyone who would step forward and take up the slack in funding? Would the Town of Nederland or the chamber of commerce (the chamber puts on the festival) put up funds to maintain their cash cow? Good thing we never got to find out. Someday, maybe.

In spite of (or perhaps because of) the rumors, the festival was gaining serious momentum. There was an opportunity to get a special postmark put on letters mailed from Nederland that week. Loveland, a plains town in Colorado, does a special remailing and postmarking of letters for Valentine's Day. It's extremely popular whether you're a philatelist or not. We had a lot of locals who got a kick out of it. Postal volume doubled that week. The Frozen but Not Dead Video Fest booked Warren Miller's *Journey* to entice in the ski crowd, who were starting to grouse at the traffic that slowed them down from getting to the town's ski area, Eldora.

Eldora was very popular with locals and folks from all over the front range because it was the closest ski resort to the Denver/Boulder metro area. When I had offices in Boulder, we'd try to finish up early on Fridays when the snow was good. We'd knock off at 3:00 p.m. and be on the slope by 4:00 p.m., when the half-priced nighttime skiing tickets kicked in. We'd ski like demons until 9:00 p.m. (a little later if we could coax the lift operator into giving us the last ride up) and then end the day at the cozy little bar at the bottom of the run with thick, rich hot chocolate laced with peppermint schnapps. Eldora is a popular place for a very good reason. Catering to the skiers a bit was good PR. The theme that year was "Party." Brent's poster was a 1950s-looking happy housewife in a party hat standing in front of an open freezer with the bearded old Grandpa figure inside. Partying and dancing were in order.

The Friday night lineup consisted mostly of the films being shown at the Backdoor Theater and Grandpa's Blue Ball at the Kathmandu Restaurant. This year, the music was provided by Shanti Groove, a "Rocky Mountain psychedelic acoustic-electric groove grass" kind of band. On Saturday night, the Yonder Mountain String Band was playing in town, too. Good "new grass" music. I had a small group for the Friday night Midnight Champagne Tour, and it went off without a hitch—without anything of note, really.

Saturday saw the parade marching off in beautiful weather. In fact, the weather had been a bit too beautiful in that it was going to be tough sledding for the Coffin Race—no snow. They had trucked in a bunch of snow from Eldora for the snow sculpturing and ended up dumping several extra loads onto the racecourse to make it a bit more challenging. When the weather cooperates, it can be fun to do snow sculptures. There were quite a few entries that inaugural year, some good and some not so good. The final winner, done by Club Ned, was a larger-than-life Gandalf with a crystal ball on his staff. A bear and Snoopy won second and third place, respectively. But the sun graced the festival that year and made it easy for the dancers before the race. A French modern dance artist by the name of Caroline Roesler did a wild interpretive dance about life and death, winding in and out of the race participants and using flowing streamers of purple silk to accentuate her moves. Then there was Dem Bones, a local kids dance troupe dressed in skeleton costumes that did a synchronized dance routine for the crowd. It was pretty artsy for the Ned fans, but it lent a little sophistication to a basic sporting event. *Games Across America*, a show on the Game Show Network, sent its announcer, Kurt Long, to emcee the race and film the whole thing for posterity and cable TV.

Two unusual additions that year promoted the freezing concept of the Frozen Dead Guy Days. One was the addition of a frozen foot bath to the Ice Queen Contest. Contestants had to sit with their feet in an ice bath while being interviewed for the position in front of the ball crowd. It made for some amusing comments from the emcee and seemed to go over well. The other was the Brain Freeze event. It was a little more difficult and resulted in some Technicolor heaves. The object was to drink as much frozen Gatorade slush as fast as you could…and survive. Both semifinalists got whopping headaches and puked their guts out, and it was declared a draw. A rough way to end the festival, but it was fun to watch.

THE PEAK YEAR

It is better to know some of the questions than all of the answers.
—James Thurber

The year 2005 turned out to be the pinnacle of the festival juggernaut. It started early in January with an e-mail sent from Belgium. It was from a producer of a show called *The Best Belgian*. The premise was that they would go around the world and enter their Belgian celebrity in contests and sporting events. Each show would feature a different place and event. The Belgian would enter, and regardless of whether he won or lost, he was probably the only (and therefore "Best") Belgian. They wanted to come to the festival and also arrange something at the shed. They wanted to set up a meeting between their representative and me before the festival to work out details and make sure that things went smoothly. I agreed, and about a week before the festival, we had that meeting at my offices in Longmont. The name of the associate producer was Malin Malin Sirrah. I had no idea even whether it was a man or a woman. It turned out to be one of the most strikingly beautiful women I've ever seen in person. One of the perks of being the Iceman, I guess.

Malin showed up at my office exactly on time, and when she stepped out of the car, I was immediately struck by her European demeanor. She was about five foot six, with blonde hair tied back in a tight little bun and beautiful blue eyes. Dressed in a tailored tweed suit that followed her every curve, when she got out of the car she walked right over to me, got just a teensy bit closer than any American does and spoke in a wonderfully different French accent: "Are you

Monsieur Beau?" I could actually hear the "eau" instead of the "o." She looked like an office model or one of "Our Man" Flint's assistants—sophisticated, beautiful and self-assured but potentially deadly. The accent and European way about her just made her more mysterious. If I had been twenty years younger and single, I'd have had my work cut out for me and would have really enjoyed my job. As it was, I decided to get to safe ground and invite her over to our house to meet my wife, since I was going to be spending a lot of time with her that weekend. My wife was expecting a foreigner with a funny name, not a Bond girl. I still had a lot of work to do, believe me.

When we got to the house, Malin was very charming and had that European air about her that just fascinates kids and is refreshing to find in rural America. She had brought little presents for all of the members of the family, and the authentic Belgian chocolates won over everybody, even my wife. Malin was very good at dealing with strangers and making them feel at ease. She was extremely efficient and laid out the plans for the video that they planned to shoot. Apparently, part of the premise of the show was that the talent wasn't aware of what exactly it was that he was entering. They would spring it on him at the last minute and get the reaction on camera. All he would know was that he was there to enter various contests in a Colorado mountain festival. We would meet at the property, and when we got to the shed, we would spring the fact on him that there was an actual dead body right there and that he was going to get close to it. I liked the concept.

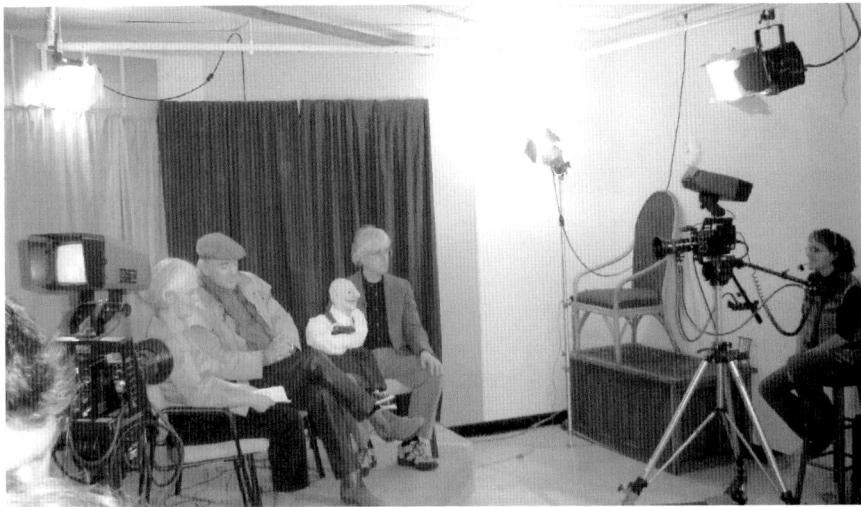

The "Best Belgian" (middle) at the CCTV54 studios in beautiful downtown Louisville.

The Peak Year

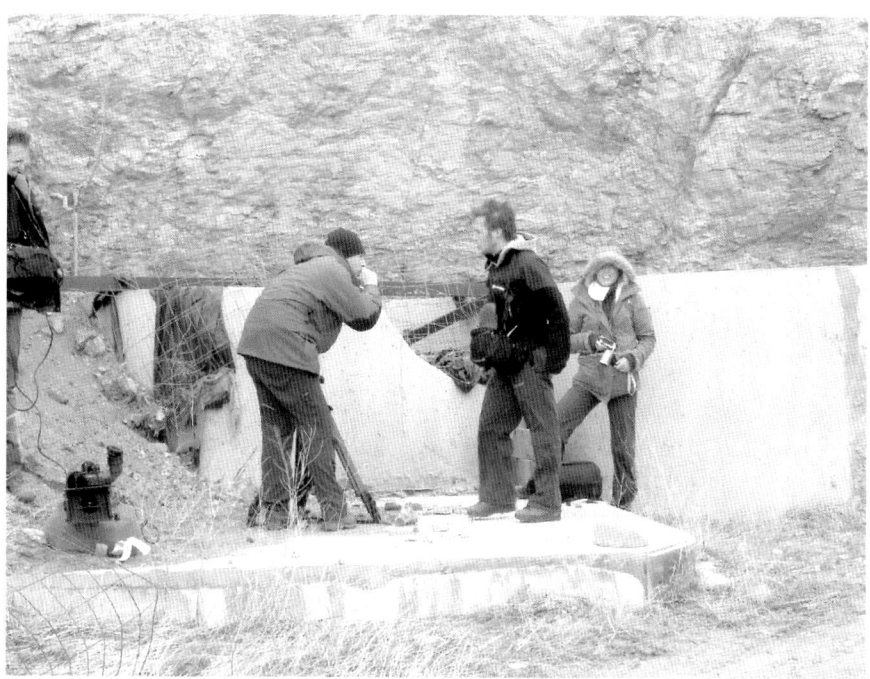

Malin, Staf and Mathias, the *Best Belgian* film crew.

I also did some PR work for them on my own. I was part of a local public access television station that did a lot of community-oriented shows. I talked to the producer of CCTV54's *East County Live!* and arranged to have the Belgian crew and a representative from the festival on the interview-formatted show that would air two days before the event. At that time, the CCTV54 studios were located in an old cable TV building next to the railroad tracks. It was small and cramped, and every time a train went by you had to stop talking for a minute or two, unless you were in the soundproof studio where they actually videotaped. They held a big open house with food and drinks, and everyone had a great time talking shop and comparing European TV with American TV—lots of technical and even social issues. Everyone who was in the know was told not to spill the beans on what the festival was all about, too. It made for some interesting conversations.

The Friday of the festival weekend, I went up early and met Malin, Herbert Flack (the "Best Belgian") and her crew. It was pretty cold and windy, but it made for some dramatic scenes with Herbert and me. When I told him that there was an actual dead body that he was going to get close to, his eyes got wide in genuine surprise. We all got a pretty good laugh out of it, not to mention that it was pretty awesome that he hadn't a clue as to what was in the shed. We shot the segment during which we talked about what contests he would enter. We had settled on the Grandpa Look-alike Contest, the Coffin Race and the Polar Plunge. I wouldn't have much to do with the race or the plunge, as I would be tied up with tours, but I agreed to help with the look-alike contest and advise him on what was the real look—Malin was going to be the makeup artist, too. We wrapped up the shoot and headed back to town.

I had a room at the old hostel in town, a couple blocks down from the motel where the Belgian contingent was staying. When they got back to their rooms, Malin and Herbert started in on his makeup for the contest that night. I made a few suggestions here and there, but mostly it was up to Malin to work some serious theatrical magic with Styrofoam, cellophane tape and styling gel. Damn, she was good! I had to get to the opening ceremonies, so I left her and went back up to the shed.

I stopped and picked up a couple of chamber members who were into running. We went up to the shed, I opened up the cryonic chamber and they dipped out a pitcher full

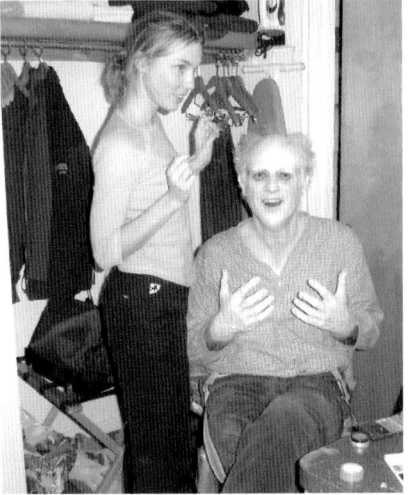

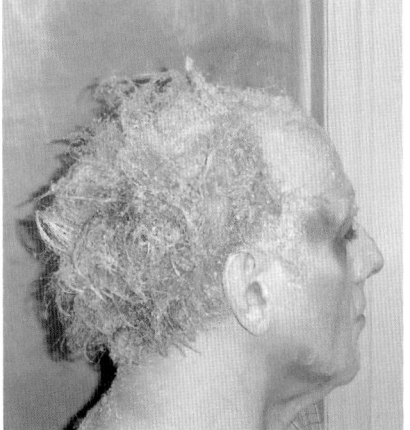

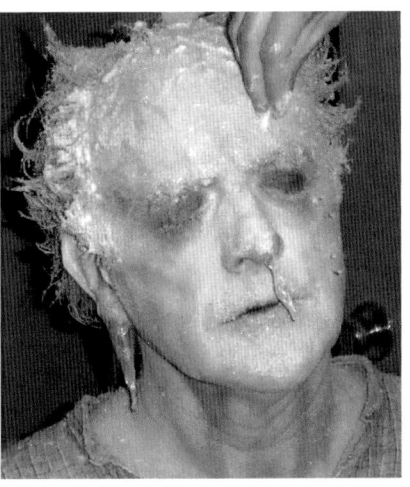

Malin helps Herbert, the "Best Belgian," with his makeup for the Grandpa Look-alike Contest, and the results. FDGD 2005.

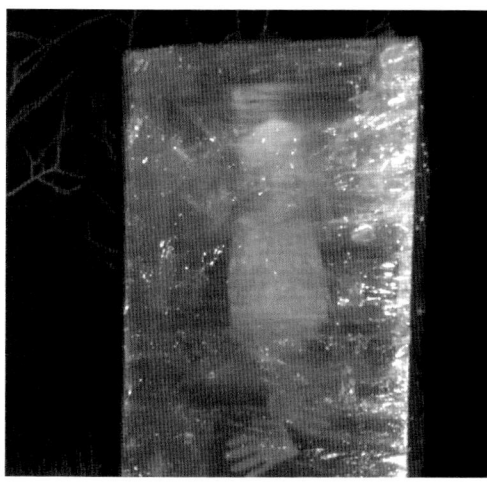

A roundabout ice sculpture in close-up, FDGD 2005.

of dry ice to carry to the opening ceremony, much like the carrying and lighting of the Olympic torch. They ran that pitcher all the way down the hill back into town and to the roundabout, where the opening ceremonies were to take place as soon as they got there. That year, the theme sculpture was a shadowy Grandpa figure in a block of ice. The figure was, of course, a dummy, and the ice block was backlit plastic wrap. We had our prerequisite skeleton dancers, and with the usual "Party with a Dead Man" blaring out over the streets of Ned, the official opening got things ramped up. I went back to my room and got ready for the ball.

We really pushed Grandpa's Blue Ball that year, among other things. There were a bunch of different art posters that year, and in fact there was some grumbling from some chamber members that they had spent too much on art. Brent made out pretty well that year, as artists went, but probably won't be truly recognized until after he dies, like all great artists. I have a personal collection of all of his posters from that year. The main poster was on the theme "It came from Cryonics," with a picture of the (by this time) iconic Grandpa with his arms stretched out like Frankenstein's monster, lower body encased in ice cubes, threatening a young man and woman. One little trivia factoid is that the artist used his son as a model for the young man. There were now almost twenty sponsors, with logos along the bottom of the poster. The

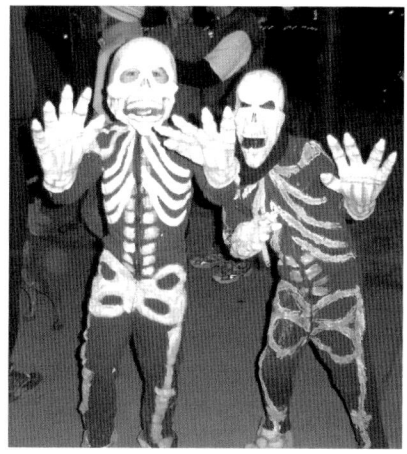

Skeleton dancers.

poster for Grandpa's Blue Ball had the iconic Grandpa figure as a swizzle stick in a high martini glass.

The ball was being held at the Black Forest Inn this year for the first time. Personally, I thought this was a bit better than the Kathmandu, which was smaller and not as high, due only in part to the Black Forest's massively steep entrance and chalet roofline. The ball was its usual self, with a kind of country/rock band, Runaway Truck Ramp. The crowd was into the band and it was pretty good. We introduced a new drink, due in part to one of our new sponsors, Rogue Brewery: Dead Guy Ale over dry ice. While it sounds good in theory, it is not so easy to do in practice. Beer tends to explode like most carbonated beverages when you drop dry ice into it. But if you wait, you can then get a doubly cold, doubly carbonated, hoppy-tasting drink that will do the job. Partway through the ball, they held the Ice Queen Contest and the Grandpa Look-alike Contest. Needless to say, the Belgian was best and walked away with the grand prize. In all the years before and since, I've never seen a Grandpa look-alike as good.

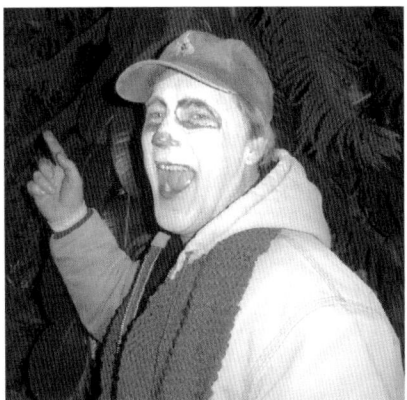

Mike, the happy ball attendee.

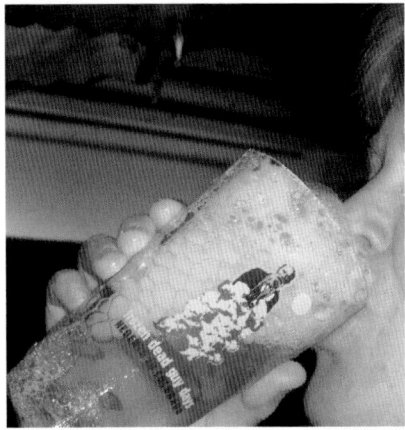

Bonnie quaffing a Dead Guy Ale over dry ice at Grandpa's Blue Ball.

The first couple of years, the contest was won by the same guy who, I have to admit, was as good as a look-alike gets until the Belgian came along. His name was Toasty, and he was sort of the town's friendly neighborhood idiot/drunk, like Otis in Mayberry. Every town has one—like how Crawford has Bush. My hometown back east had its own guy, named Drifty. Everybody knew him and took care of him when he was incapable of taking care of himself, which was most Friday and Saturday nights. It also just so happened that Toasty was a dead ringer for the iconic picture of the frozen dead guy, sunken eyes, beard and all. A little

The Peak Year

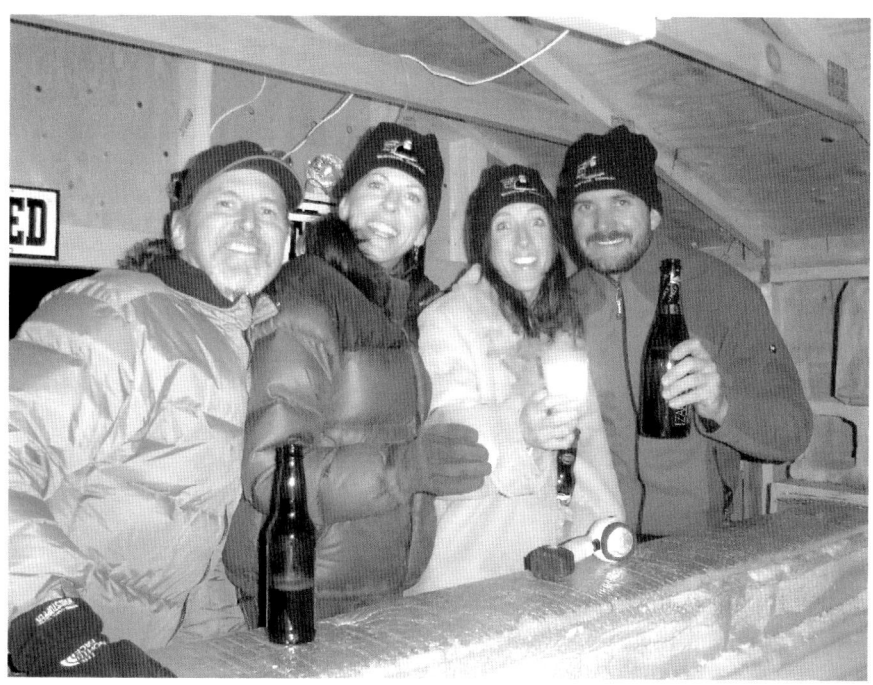

Midnight Champagne Tour, FDGD 2005.

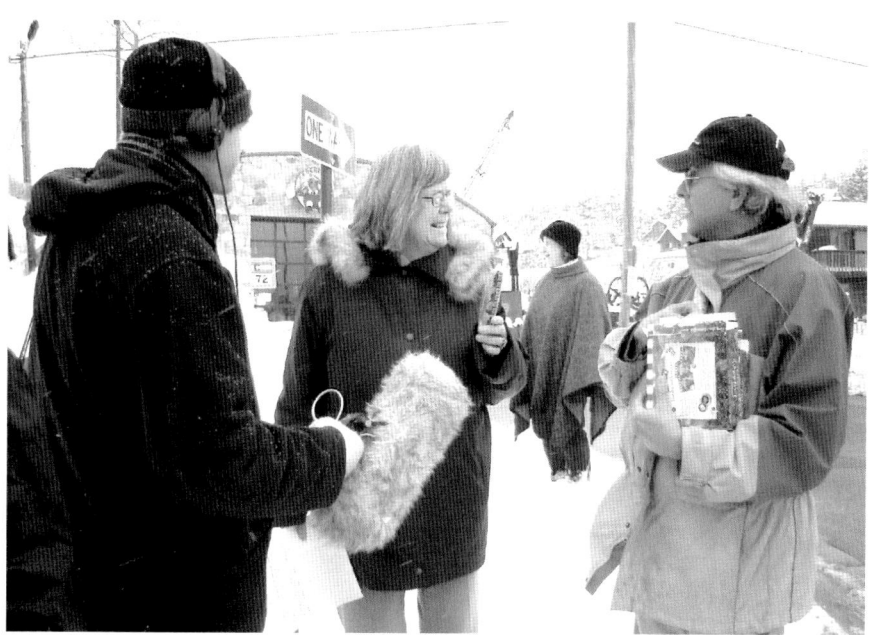

Aud and Brent at the roundabout, FDGD 2005.

makeup and a couple of props, and it was easy to see how he had won the contest in prior years. But the Belgian changed that, and deservedly so.

The Midnight Champagne Tour was small that year. Two of the volunteers who worked their butts off asked to go, and they brought their significant others. That was it. The five of us hung in the 'hood with Grandpa for a while and did a little toasting. Then, since everyone was beat from the long day, I took them all back to town and dropped them off. It was almost 2:00 a.m., but I had no desire to go back to the hostel and maybe run into Aud.

Aud Morstoel, daughter of Bredo Morstoel himself, was in town to be the parade's grand marshal. The chamber of commerce, in a moment of what later turned out to be insanity, decided that it would be a good thing to invite Trygve's mother, Aud, over from Norway to be grand marshal of the parade. Aud had gone back to Norway a short time after Trygve was deported and had been living with Tryg in Oslo ever since. Her decision to leave back then was brought about by a little brush with the law. She walked out on a judge in a courtroom during her hearing, and they were contemplating contempt charges. She reached a mutual agreement with them and left the country. Now, ten years later, she was back as a visiting celebrity. This would probably have worked out better if not for Aud's, uh, condition.

Aud was in great physical condition but had some psychological problems. She was on medication, and Trygve usually kept a tight rein on her. She was prone to abusive outbreaks, but that may have just been due to her basic personality...or the booze. She was fine as long as she was regulated and they kept her away from the alcohol. Trygve had lined up a Norwegian radio announcer to fly with Aud and chaperone her to Nederland. They got through all right, but the fatal crack in the wall started at customs when they confiscated Aud's meds. In retrospect, it was like watching one of those disaster flicks where a tiny thing that ends up causing catastrophic damage has already occurred, but everybody is unaware and just parties on—like the faulty electrical box in *Towering Inferno*. By the time I got to Ned on Friday, she had already been off her meds for almost a week, had brushed off the "chaperone" and was starting to be a regular at the Pioneer Inn (PI) and the Black Forest (Ned's foremost watering holes). I didn't want to deal with her, and so I drove around town looking for something to do.

At a time when most people are ready for bed, I have an unusual metabolic thing that kicks in. Once I get past midnight, no matter how long the day, I usually get this burst of energy and have trouble winding down for several hours. I've done some of my best work in the wee hours of the morning, and at times when I'm left to my own devices, I tend to gravitate to working until sunrise and then sleeping until after noon. I am not a morning person, as most people think of them, although I accomplish a lot of things in the morning before most people are awake. I had a partner once who was a real morning person. He'd wake up at about 5:00 a.m., we'd get together for breakfast/bedtime snack and I'd let him know all of the things that I'd worked on overnight. I'd go to bed, and he'd head out and take care of all of the business I'd set up. We'd pass again about twelve hours later, roles reversed, and I would finish up any unfinished business he had left as he headed to supper and early bedtime. The two of us ran a twenty-four-hour service that way. So when I was in Nederland at 2:00 a.m. and they had rolled in the streets, even on a festival night, I had tons of energy and went looking for something to do.

Ned at night is kind of a spooky place. The police had told all of the business owners in Ned that there was no way that they could cover all of them for burglaries. They suggested that everyone leave their lights on so that the few patrols there were could see into the shops and hopefully deter crime. The upshot of this is that it's two o'clock in the morning, the whole town is lit up and there's not a soul in sight. It's like driving through a town where everybody just up and disappeared one night. The roundabout was lit up, and Grandpa's dimly glowing ice cube looked out over the empty streets. I didn't find a soul until I stumbled upon the ice sculpture tent.

This year we had brought back an event from the previous year and added a little to it. In 2004, we had various artists sculpt piles of snow around town. It was difficult due to the weather that year being unseasonably warm. This year they had erected a huge tent, had brought the snow in and had packed it into several different blocks, all available to the public for whatever free-form sculpture they wanted. It was a great thing to get whole families involved during the day—or a bunch of drunks late at night. When I pulled up, there were four or five guys standing inside the huge tent, out of the little breeze that had started to blow. They had the remains of a twelve-pack and were just standing around talking and shivering.

It was a little dark inside, as they had turned off the electricity to the tent for the night, so no one could see very well. The tent had clear windows, so some light from the streetlights outside did come through. Everyone was gathered around the big spot of light like it was a campfire. I came up to the group and started to chat with them. When I told them who I was, they all got a big kick out of it, and we started to discuss things like death and dying. We exchanged intoxicants, my joint for their beer, and I said that I had a boombox in the truck with some cool music, if they were interested.

Colorado's Iceman

Back in '02, I had run for sheriff of Boulder County. I was a real underdog, but I ended up getting over 20 percent of the vote. Not bad for a libertarian. One of my fellow candidates, running for coroner, was a music mixologist on the side. Dr. Reptile was his moniker, and he had made me a special CD called *Dead and Dying, the Coroner's Race in Boulder County*. It was a collection of songs that all mentioned death or dying. Naturally, it started with Oingo Boingo's "Party with a Dead Man," but it also had such eclectic tunes as "Dead Skunk in the Middle of the Road" by Louden Wainright, John Prine's "Please Don't Bury Me," the Stones' "Dead Flowers" and Warren Zevon's "Things to Do in Denver When You're Dead." Every time I listen to the twenty-five songs on that disc, I can't help but get in the mood. I was lamenting that we couldn't turn it up too loud because it was on battery power when one of the guys came over and said that he could take care of that. Turns out that he was one of the main Public Works guys in Ned and had set up most of the tents and electric odds and ends himself. He went outside for a minute, and when he came back, he plugged in a couple of lights and a heater, as well as the boombox. We were stylin' now!

T (the Public Works guy) said that he was up for a little sculpting, but everyone else was petering out. They left, and T and I started to design a possible sculpture. We broke out the pipe weed and, after a few inspiring bowls, went to work. There were several sculptures already started, the most impressive being the Loch Ned Mermaid. She was a lovely, buxom beauty, ten feet tall sitting on a casket. Her tresses, in wonderfully detailed curls, fell along her shoulders and breasts like the waves of the ocean. It was so good that it was actually what inspired us to make our own attempt. Snow sculptures are very zen. Such effort to create such temporary beauty, like a Picasso scratched in the sand at low tide—something to be appreciated in its ephemeral existence, as well as its artistic merits.

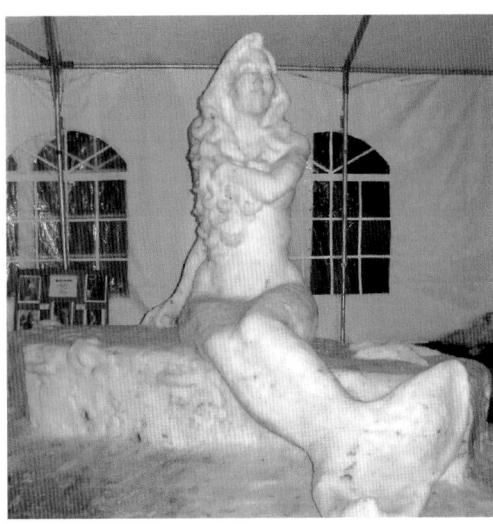

The first-place ice sculpture, FDGD 2005.

T and I decided to do a sculpture of the frozen dead guy himself, which seemed

The Peak Year

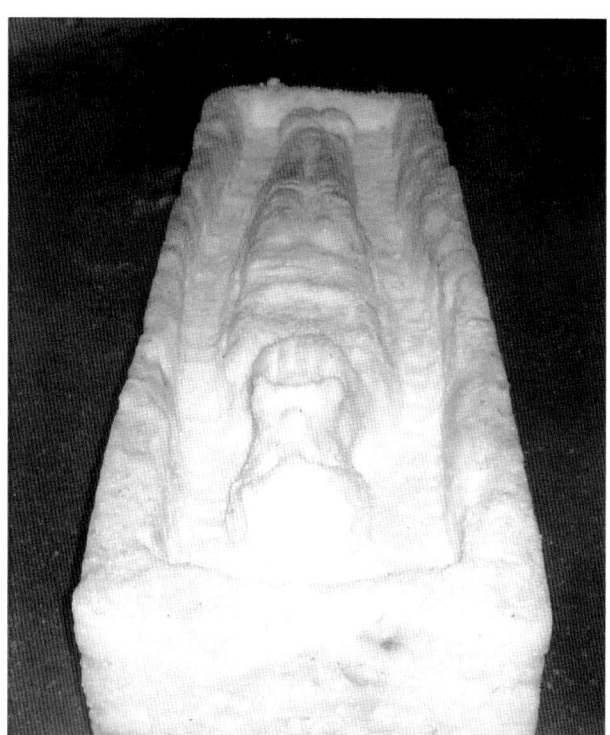

Left: T and Bo's third-place ice sculpture, FDGD 2005.

Below: Snow sculptures at the 2005 FDGD.

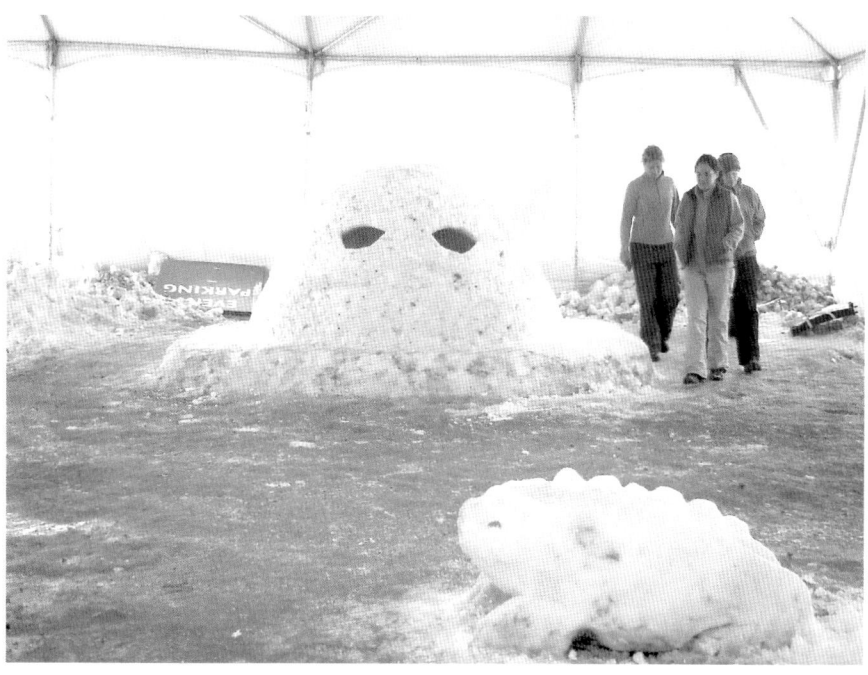

the appropriate thing to do considering that I was one of the sculptors. Considering that we only had my Swiss army knife and a couple of plastic cups, I think we did a fairly good representation of the old guy. All I know is that we had a blast jivin' to the dead music and carving up the dead snow into a dead guy. It must not have been too bad of an effort since we ended up winning third place. We hung out in the tent until about four o'clock in the morning, with the wind picking up to the point that we couldn't hear the music. After the third or fourth time through, the CD was getting a little tiresome anyway, so we finished up and dropped off the entry form, and I took T home. We promised to get together the next night, but I never saw him again until the next year's festival, which is another tale.

Saturday morning came and I took up the first tour. We had not scheduled a midmorning tour so that I might be able to make it to the parade. I came back down after a little problem (see the "Notes on Ned" chapter) and got lined up in the parade with everyone. I was right behind a half-dozen big hairy guys dressed in flamingo-pink tutus and carrying a flamingo-themed coffin. They were the Manitou-tus. There was a bit of a rivalry going on between Nederland and Manitou Springs, a small town near Colorado Springs, due to a celebration that they hold there every year that also includes a Coffin Race. Apparently, their patron was a female miner who—whether alive or dead—went down a big hill in a coffin and "saved the day" back in the old mining days. The modern version (so I'm told; I was invited to race one year, but discretion being the better part of valor, I declined) is something like a four-wheel-drive soapbox derby down a mining tailings slope. They also have six-man teams. Ever since the principals of their race had heard about ours, they had sent a team, and the people of Ned usually fielded one back. Their race was held in the fall, and ours was in the spring, so it worked out well—lots of time to hype the thing all year long.

Driving in a parade up the main drag of Ned in my red, white and blue pickup truck, following cross-dressers in pink tutus, throwing dry ice pellets out of the window to the howls of all the kids—not an everyday experience altogether. Although the thing with the kids is to be expected. Kids and dry ice have a natural attraction for each other. When my kids were younger, I'd bring home pieces of dry ice after the ice runs, and we'd play with them in the kitchen. Did you know that sippy cups make great things to blow up with dry ice? With the spout lid, they turn into fog machines or carbon dioxide–powered squirt guns. With the travel lid on they turn into (relatively) harmless time bombs. The pressure will blow the lid off within a few seconds (longer with less ice) at a reasonably low pressure but will blow it twenty feet

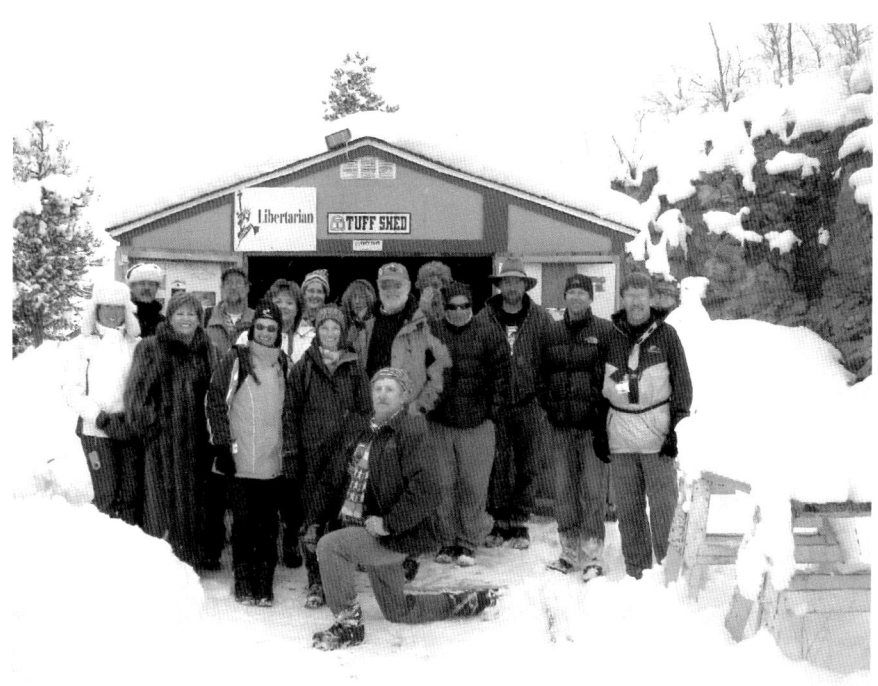

Above: Bo and a big tour, FDGD 2005.

Below: A tour guide opening the shed for the tour, FDGD 2005.

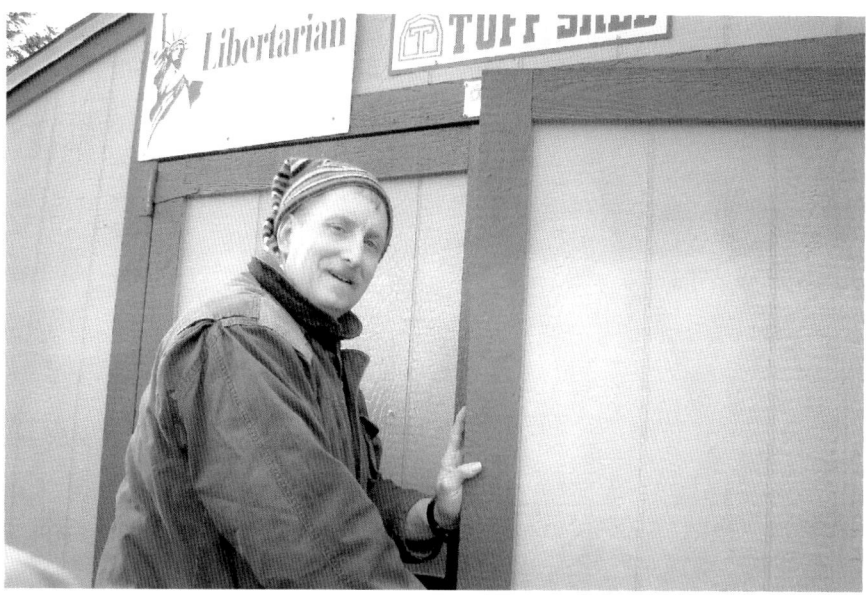

up in the air with a magnificent *pop*! Waiting for it to blow produced many a giggle. It also taught respect for hard, flying objects and served as an intro to explosives and how to handle them.

Home school has such wonderful subjects. But I would also bring the dry ice dog and pony show to schools and academies all over the front range. I have given many lectures and seminars on the frozen dead guy and dry ice. Grandpa gets their attention, and the dry ice keeps it and makes them think. Of course, I learn something once in a while, too—like when I talked to a seventh-grade class in Gilpin County. The boys (the girls just watched) showed me that you really could eat dry ice and live to tell the tale. They would crunch it up, swallow it and burp little clouds of fog. I wouldn't recommend it to anyone with fillings, but it's possible. From them I developed a technique to put a piece between my front teeth and exhale over it—it looks like dragon's breath. It can "burn" you if you hang on to it for too long, but keeping it moving around whether in your mouth or in your hand is the key to enjoying it and not getting burned.

Fun and games with dry ice. Throwing pellets of dry ice out the window and dropping them into outstretched, gloved hands was no big thing for me. I saw it as an opportunity for more people to learn about the wonders of frozen carbon dioxide. Naturally, someone complained about the potential for the possibility of someone getting the tiniest bit hurt, and so I was told to not to throw any ice anymore. Sad.

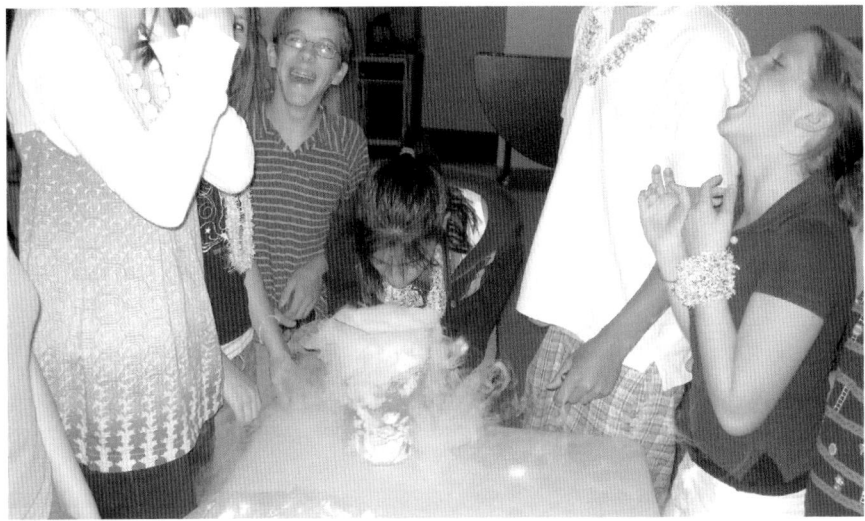

Teaching kids about the fun parts of science at the dry ice seminars.

The parade finished up, and I went back to doing tours for the rest of the day. I had settled into a routine, polished after four years of repetition, that I could pretty much do in my sleep. When the tour group would arrive, I'd greet them outside the main building and point out various items of interest lying around. Then we'd go inside, and I'd give a little spiel on what was in there, and then we'd all go to the shed. Once in a while, I'd reverse the order to give the rubes what they want and then hit them with the hook and jerk their dough. That was something I learned at my granddaddy's knee. He was an old carney worker from before the war. There are still the occasional strange words that sneak into my vocabulary as a legacy from him: calling bread "punk," your watch your "super" and an overcoat a "Bennie," after Jack Benny's coat. He also taught me the classic carney rule: there's one born every minute, and it might as well be you who takes advantage of it. Of course, growing up in the Depression may have had something to do with his attitude, too. So, in light of my grandfather's sage advice, I had created a little souvenir stand to go with our freaky little sideshow. Step right up, folks! Grab yourself a little piece of history in the making! We got gen-u-ine frozen dead guy shed pieces, with serial numbers and a certificate of authenticity signed by the man himself! We got pictures…we got autographed Dead Guy hats…we got Wizbalm…we got Dead Guy brownies…we got just what you need!

Yeah, I went hog-wild with the prospect of selling souvenirs and put out quite a display. The shed pieces were from the original metal shed that we took down to put up the Tuff Shed. I had kept the sliding doors to it, cut one into small pieces and stamped a serial number in the corner of each. I made up a really nice-looking certificate of authenticity and printed it out on certificate paper. I got gold seals and a stamp, and when you got one, you got your name included on a list of benefactors, which is kept with Grandpa until he is reanimated, so he'll know who his friends are. I was asking twenty-five dollars for a piece of history that cost me twenty-five cents. My Grampy would have been proud. Rogue Brewery, one of our sponsors, had donated a bunch of its black hats with "Dead Guy" on them, referring to Dead Guy Ale. I offered to autograph them for people for a "small donation." There are a few people out there who own a genuine Dead Guy hat with the Iceman's autograph. Lucky them. There are at least a dozen people with pieces of Bredo's original home, including Bill Geist, who actually has two, if he ever finds the one he lost.

In the picture of one of the Sunday tourists proudly holding his shed piece, you might notice that there's a foot of snow in the background. You might

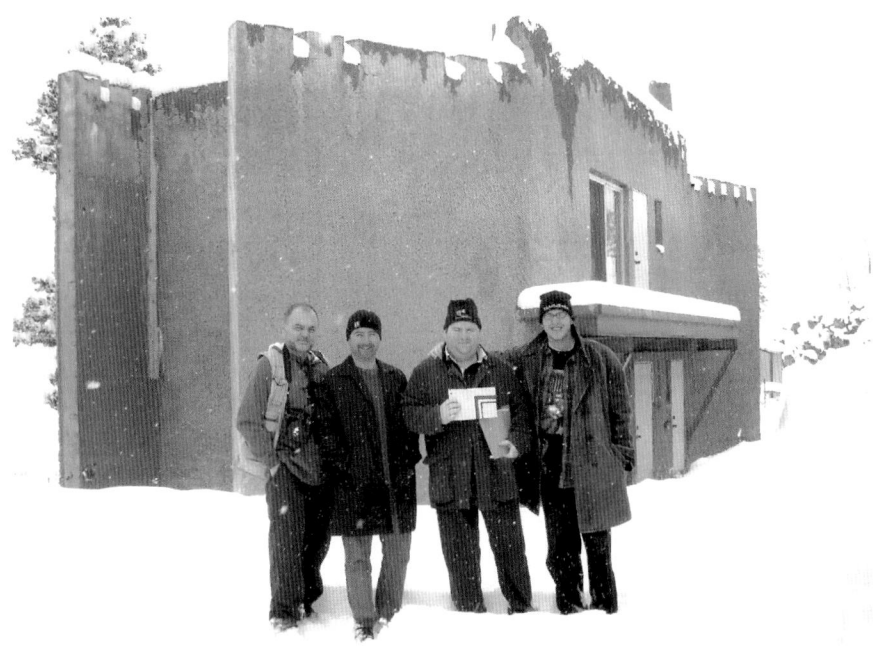

A tourist proudly displays his certified shed piece, FDGD 2005.

also notice that the parade pictures from Saturday were taken on a bright, sunny, warm day with no snow in sight. After a day and a half of nonstop festival activities in a typical spring warm spell, a typical spring blizzard blew in that night and dumped a foot of snow. Yesiree! If you don't like the weather in Colorado, wait a day…it'll change. Seventy degrees Saturday and a high of twenty on Sunday. Late Saturday night, everybody was walking home from Grandpa's Crawl in new-fallen snow. It seemed to finally put a little damper on the frenzy that typified the first two days. I drove around for a while again, just enjoying the snow and quiet and trying to remember more of "Stopping by Woods on a Snowy Evening," Robert Frost's beautiful ode to a snowstorm. I had a good time working out new words to "Stopping by Dead Guy on a Snowy Evening," and maybe someday I will include it in a Dead Guy poetry collection. The before and after pictures are pretty good though. Fortunately, I did not have miles to go before I slept. I had to go back to the hostel and Aud.

Not much else happened that Sunday, with the storm keeping people away and everybody digging out. But that crack in the wall was about to widen. Aud decided that she didn't want to leave right away, since she was

THE PEAK YEAR

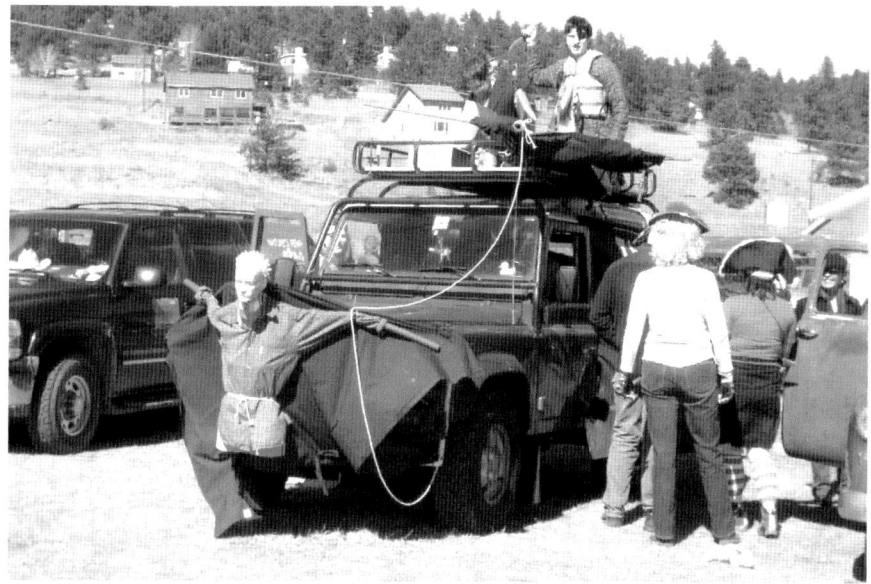

A pirate float in the parade the day before it snowed.

having such a good time. She decided to continue to stay at the hostel. Now, the hostel was really defunct. A developer had just bought it and closed it down but hadn't started renovations yet. He had offered it to the chamber to house any dignitaries coming to the festival. Aud, the radio reporter and I all stayed there. The reporter left Monday, but Aud wouldn't leave. She stayed for several weeks but had to leave after the "incident" and ended up in an apartment in Boulder. But I'm getting ahead of myself.

In the weeks following the festival, everyone started putting pressure on Aud to leave, but she was more interested in having a good time. An alcoholic, off her meds, with a pocketful of money and a free place to live, she was in her glory. She was drinking every day, and there were times when the owner of the Black Forest thought for sure that he'd be calling the ambulance or something when she tried to go down his steps in the snow. The Black Forest steps are deadly. Thirty feet high and steep. When they're covered in snow, they can be deceptive. Aud never fell far, probably due to her experience with snow in Norway, but she slipped often enough to give everyone at the bar a heart attack. Aud was bar hopping and each day was buzzed just a little bit earlier. Everyone was trying to get her to leave.

At one point, Theresa, the head of the chamber, called Trygve and tried to get him to talk to his mother. She apparently mentioned that Aud's hygiene was suffering, but by the time it got back to Aud, it was translated more like, "Yo mama stinks!" One night, Theresa and her husband were in a Ned restaurant, and Aud came in with a snoot full and laid into Theresa about the phone call to her son. At one point, Aud actually hit Theresa in front of lots of witnesses. Theresa, kind person that she is, refused to press any charges, realizing that it was the booze talking. That was all well and good until the next morning, when Aud came into Theresa's store buzzed already and lit into her again in front of customers. There was nothing Theresa could do except call the cops and get her taken out. Then, due to the nature of the legal system, Theresa pressed the issue in the restaurant the night before, when Aud had hit her in front of witnesses. Easier to get a case for assault in public than trespass in a storefront.

Naturally, this infuriated both Aud and Trygve. Trygve was a dutiful son, but he did his mother no favors by trying to cover up her problems. But he's fifty years old, and they still live together, so I guess I can see his point of view. I wouldn't piss off my mother over such a thing if I lived with her, either. There were a lot of transatlantic calls and discussions with lawyers and the INS (remember the last time Aud was in town?). Aud moved down from Ned into an apartment in Boulder while she was waiting for the courts. Trygve called me one day and asked me to move a mattress for his mom from Ned to Boulder. I picked it up and brought it to her, and when I got to her apartment, she went inside and made a phone call.

She got Tryg on the phone, and they started to yell at each other in Norwegian. She handed the phone to me, and Tryg started in on me about Theresa and Nederland and how his poor old mother had never done anything wrong and how they were persecuting her; he threatened to shut down the whole festival if they didn't drop all charges and apologize to his mother and him. And then Aud went off on me, personally. If you've never heard a Norwegian argument or never been cursed at in Norwegian, you've missed a treat. Their language is very melodic and high pitched and wavers around in a singsong fashion. It's tough to believe that they are actually that angry. Aud was hard to take seriously until she picked up that broomstick and started to get physical. I pulled a strategic retreat. That was the last time I ever saw Aud.

Eventually, everyone reached an agreement that Aud would leave, and they'd drop the charges. Trygve called me finally and started to say how it proved that she was innocent because they had to let her go. I told him no, that they said they wouldn't press the charges if she left the country and didn't come back. She's pretty much banned from this country. "Not unlike yourself," I said. He didn't have much to say after that. Way back in 2001, before 9/11, Trygve had told me that he was ready to come back to America as soon as they made the borders between the EU and America free and open. God bless ya Tryg; you're a dyed-in-the-wool libertarian. You stood up for your principles and it got you deported. But, now you're thinking that you'll get free and open borders here in the United States with the borders closed up after the terrorists bombed the Twin Towers? Not bloody likely. Sending Aud over didn't work out too well, either. Now she's persona non grata.

Trygve thought that he could control the festival. His threats to discontinue it were empty, because the entire festival was under the control and auspices of the chamber of commerce. He did garner a little support from people in Nederland who thought that if he wasn't behind it the festival shouldn't happen. Fortunately, that was a very small if vocal minority. Trygve could, however, control his own property. He refused to allow any more tours, and for the next several years there were no official tours during the festival.

THE LATER YEARS

In 2006, the festival was a bit off due to there being no tours. But there were plenty of other things to do, and we all just adapted. I did take a group of reporters up to the shed right before the festival. Two Norwegians, Knut and Silje of the Norwegian Press Corps, had come to Ned just to cover the hometown boy's festival for the folks back in Norway. I took them and Pat from Central City's newspaper, the *Register Call*, up to try and get a little publicity going. Instead of tours during the festival, I was giving a lecture at the "FDGD Expo Center," otherwise known as the Best Western Lodge. They were also showing the recently revamped *Grandpa's Still in the Tuff Shed* and had a lecture from the real cryonics folks, all sandwiched in between my lectures. Then I gave a traveling lecture, as it were, at the FDG mausoleum. This was a specially built Tuff Shed that had been made to look like a mausoleum wall, with crypts and a marble surface and everything. The sides drop down, and for some of the early festivals, the coffin racecourse ran right through it. It was a busy time, information wise.

The Blue Ball had an Afro-Latin jazz band playing, which was different and probably not quite as appreciated as the usual country/rock-oriented bands from the past. Ned is a mountain town, and the residents' tastes tend to run more along the lines of Willie Nelson than Santana. The ball was enjoyable but not memorable. Some people had a really good time. There were a lot of different things that year. A yoga instructor gave classes on the Corpse pose. Bizung Family African Drummers were at the Coffin Race and the Polar Plunge. Pamalla Stockho, author of *One Too Many Frozen Dead*

FROZEN DEAD GUY DAYS 2006

presents

"CRONICLES OF THE ICE MAN"

Running a backyard cryonic facility for fun and profit

Told by: **BO SHAFFER**, "the ice man"

DAY_____TIME_____

$5 adults - $3 kids

ADMIT ONE

A ticket for the first presentation of the chronicles at the 2005 FDGD.

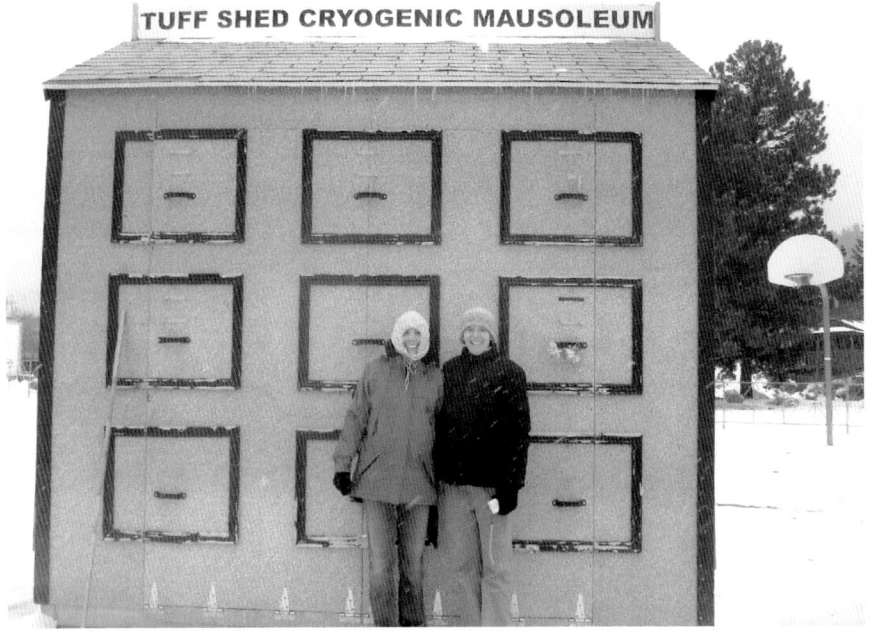

Two attendees at the chronicles lecture given at the Tuff Shed mausoleum.

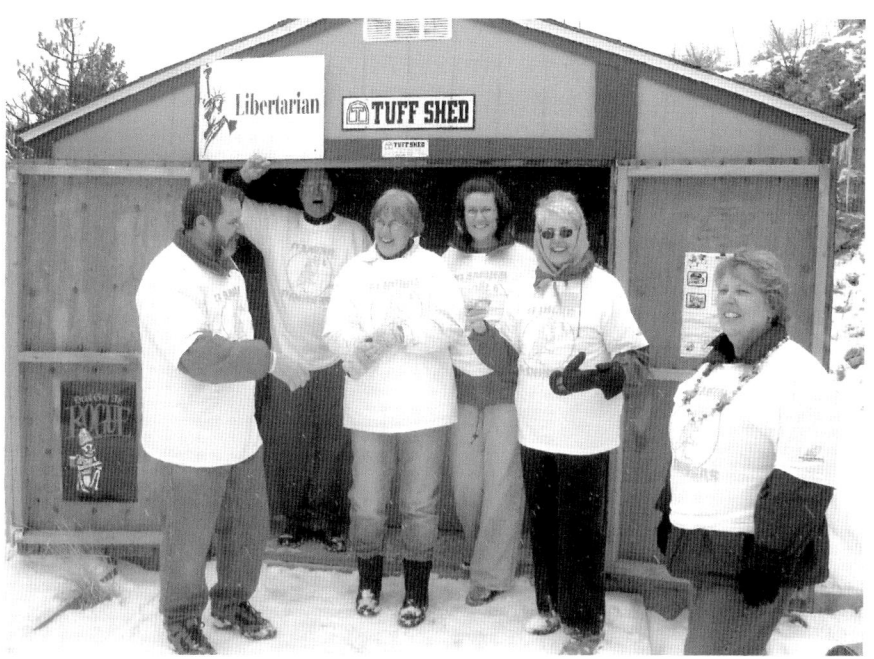

The Flaming Flamingo tour, FDGD 2006.

Guys, did a book signing. I had consulted with her while she wrote a mystery that was essentially the Iceman finding a recently murdered body in the Tuff Shed cryonic chamber with Grandpa and all the fun that results from that. At the ball, they even had an auction where all sorts of dead-related things were auctioned off to the macabre.

The only tour I did that year was a special one for the Flaming Flamingoes. This is a group of semiretired people who gather together and go on mini trips, but they never know where until they get there. The president makes it up and is the only one who knows all of the details. They came on a four-hour bus ride and were pretty amazed when they found that they were at Frozen Dead Guy Days. Then, when they got a special dispensation to go to the shed when tours had been cancelled, it just made their day. We had fun at the shed.

In 2007, the festival was pretty surreal for me. Everything was crammed into the first twenty-four hours. I had two film crews, one from the Smithsonian (also doing bits for *National Geographic*) and another from England. I had gone to Denver early and done some errands, as well as picked up some extra dry

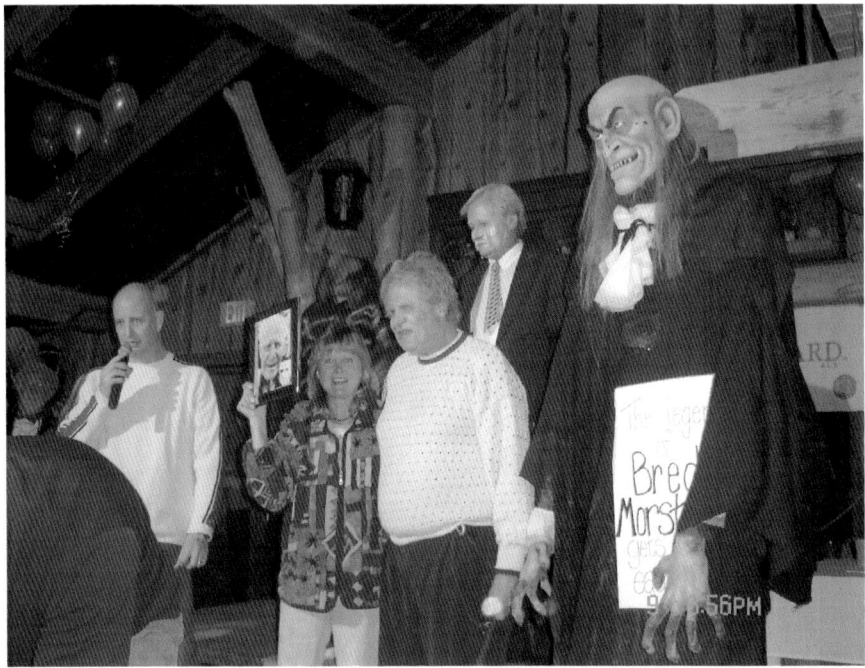

The Grandpa Look-alike Contest, with Cousin It way in the back.

ice for the festival. I got to Ned and took the film crews up to the facility. We shot some footage and then headed back to the opening ceremony at the roundabout. There were the usual skeleton dancers and the obligatory Oingo Boingo tune. These dancers were kind of cute, though, with feather boas and tight outfits. Then we broke up, and everyone headed out to get ready for the Blue Ball.

One of the best balls ever started off with the Ice Queen Contest. There were quite a few entries, some scary, some sexy. People in Nederland get cabin fever in the winter, and sex seems to occupy their minds a lot then. The final contestant, who ended up winning, flashed the judges and audience with pretty hot knickers. Sort of like Sparkle Farkle of the Farkle family, for those old enough to remember *Laugh-In*. The Grandpa Look-alike Contest was sort of anticlimactic after that. The guys were mostly into the dead part of the frozen dead guy look-alike contest. There was one last-minute entry who looked a lot like Cousin It from the Addams family—turned out to be the band leader.

I had never met Vince Herman. I had heard about him, though—frontman for Leftover Salmon, one of Boulder's premier bands. He was playing that night with his new band, Great American Taxi, and they had sent word that they needed some dry ice for their show. I showed up backstage, which at the Black Forest is outside, and met Vince and his band, complete with roadies and techies. They needed the dry ice to charge their fog machine, which would be used to resurrect the frozen dead Iron Man. I got talking to a couple of the techies and one of the band members, and I offered to help. We stood around for a few minutes, discussed things and shared some smokes and a few pieces of mold and then got right to work. We really got into wrapping Vince up in layers of aluminum foil and knocking him back down on the cart every time he sat up and wanted another drink or a hit off that smoke going around. Then they loaded their equipment on the cart, and the rest of the band, dressed as doctors, wheeled him into the ballroom and started the show. They started up strobe lights and colored spots and gave a little spiel about resurrecting the dead. Then they started up the fog machine, and billowing clouds of dry ice fog were everywhere. The crowd was diggin' it. The strobes got faster as Vince started to sit up and tear the foil from around himself like a big frozen TV dinner. The lights were flashing, people were yelling and Vince grabbed a strategically placed guitar and opened up with the first notes of Black Sabbath's "Iron Man"… and the crowd went wild. They played for hours, and the place was a frenzy of dancing, staggering males and females doing the things they love to do. The place was a wreck by the time they finished, but it sure was a good time.

I was feeling pretty energetic, so after helping the band pack the truck and sending them off in grand style, I went back inside and cleaned up a little.

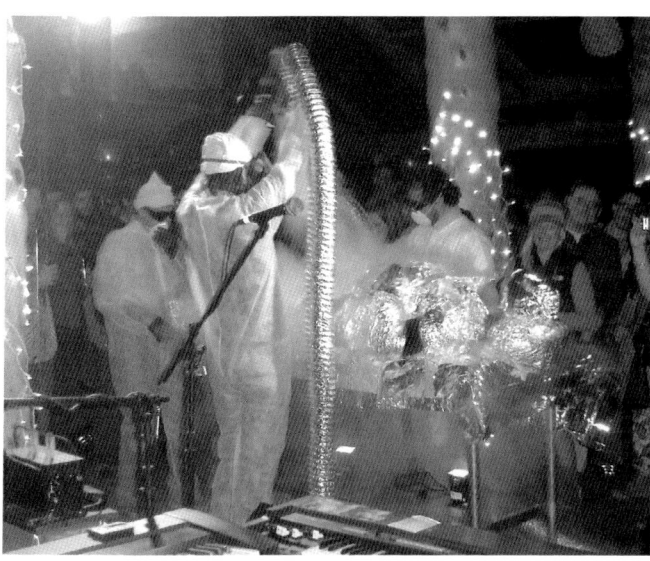

Great American Taxi resurrecting Vince at the Blue Ball.

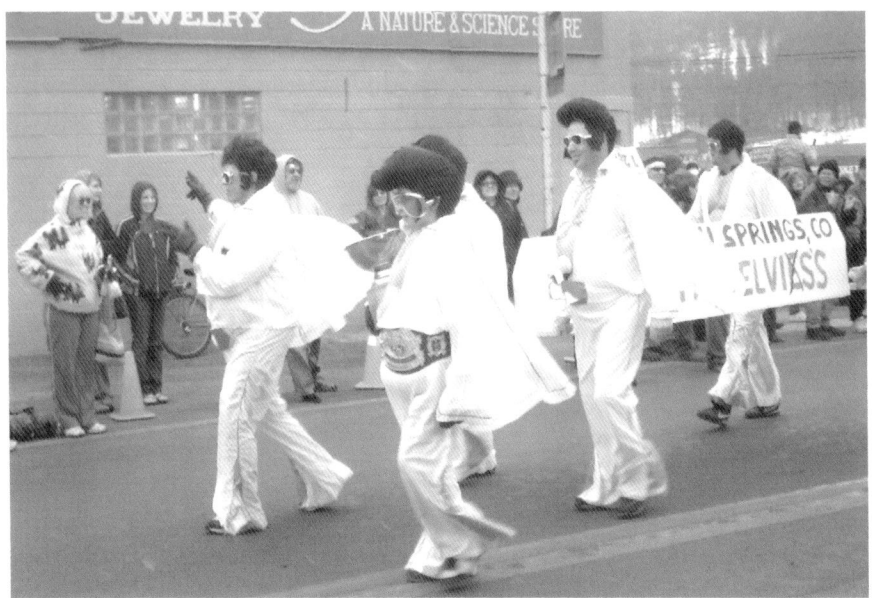
Manitou Springs' entry in the yearly Coffin Race rivalry, the Dead Elvises.

That's when I found Vince's computer that he had left in a corner, and so I left to look for him. I drove around town for a while and never did find him that night (I did later, and when I returned the computer to him he was really grateful), but I did pick up a couple of drunks. There's a whole long story about these two drunks up on my FDGD website for 2007—Chadwick the Third and Doctor Ron. Ned late at night is certainly an unusual place.

The next day, the weather was fairly atrocious, with snow and blowing snow. The Smithsonian crew couldn't even shoot the Coffin Race because their equipment got too wet. The parade was short, but the usual suspects were there. Zack and his evil secret society that punishes the stupid, SORP, with its batwinged, flame-throwing hearse, complete with a couple of hearse wenches—always a hit. The Manitou Coffin Race team this year was the Dead Elvises—Elvii?—six big guys in late-career Elvis suits, beer bellies and all. The rivalry goes on. It was snowing like a dog on the Polar Plunge, and you could barely see the contestants from where you had to stand. It didn't snow all that much, but it was a fitting white and quiet end to a colorful and wild couple of days.

The Later Years

In 2008, the festival started off with a party atmosphere. The ice sculpture in the roundabout was a giant face of Grandpa blowing the foam off a tall, frosty mug of beer. Great colors, too. The ball had Ukulele Loki and his Gadabout Dead Guy Orchestra. It included a real live burlesque act and was reminiscent of how a party might have been a hundred years ago. Pretty impressive show. The ball was held back in the renovated old gymnasium of the community center. The volunteers had made some pretty wild light and fabric sculptures to decorate the ball, and it was very surreal. And then came the Ice Queen Contest.

All of the contestants were pretty smoking in their festive snow outfits. There were feather boas, slinky metallic dresses and outlandish fashion wigs. To tell the truth, I don't really remember what most of them looked like that much, because when the emcee asked the audience which one they liked the best, the number one contestant—who was dressed in a frilly bunch of pretty skirts and a tight tube top with a bright blue wig (à la Uma Thurman in *Pulp Fiction*)—turned around and flipped up her skirts. She was buck naked underneath. There was an instant of jaw dropping and then wild applause, as the contest observers were mostly male. All of the other contestants faded into the background as she repeated the gesture a couple of times. She won hands down.

The parade was in nice weather again, and there were some really imaginative groups, not just Coffin Race entrants. A zombie dance troupe you could understand, but alpacas? Hey, don't be frozen—wear alpaca! Flying monkeys, flying pigs, politicians, Girl Scouts…a very eclectic group of Coffin Racers that year. The zombie dancers did a couple of routines and were actually quite entertaining. Good timing.

The biggest highlight of that year was the one and only tour. I had been contacted by some law enforcement people who knew me from my run for sheriff. There was a large local company that was started in Boulder years ago by some former Boulder sheriff deputies but grew to be nationwide. It was on the cutting edge of security and emergency services. One of the big wheels of the company was going to be in town, and he was a fan and wanted to see the festival and do a tour of the shed. He only had a couple of hours in his high-powered executive schedule, and I said that this might not be enough time to get up from Boulder, do the tour and get back down to the Denver airport. The guy said that wouldn't be a problem. On Saturday afternoon, a big black executive helicopter came up the canyon and landed by the reservoir where the flights for life usually land. The executive and his entourage disembarked, and a couple of black

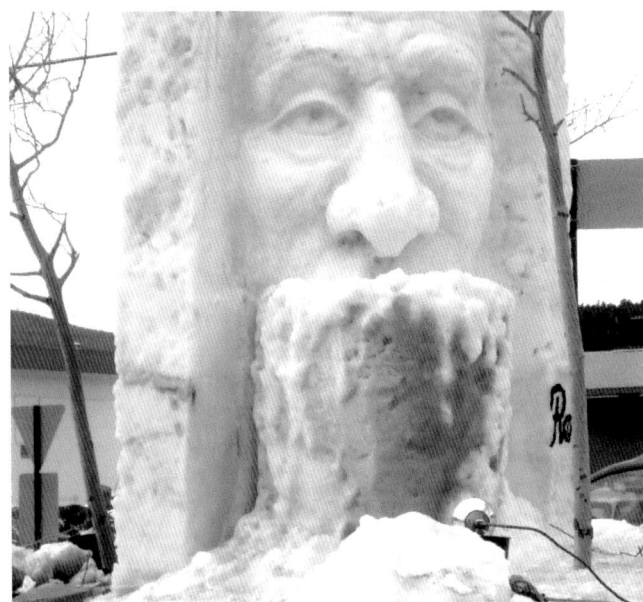

A roundabout ice sculpture for the 2008 FDGD.

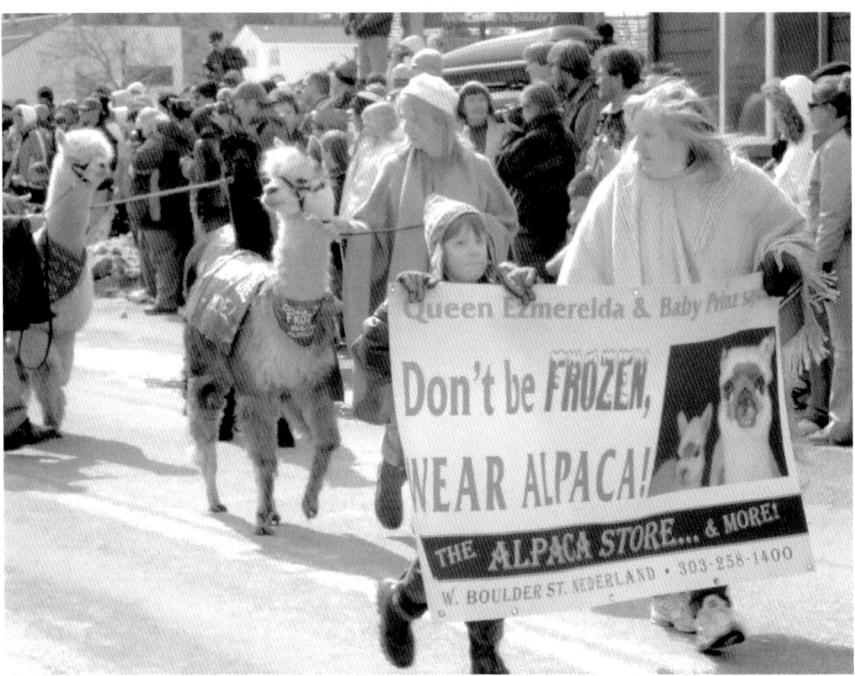

Even animals get into the 2008 FDGD fun.

THE LATER YEARS

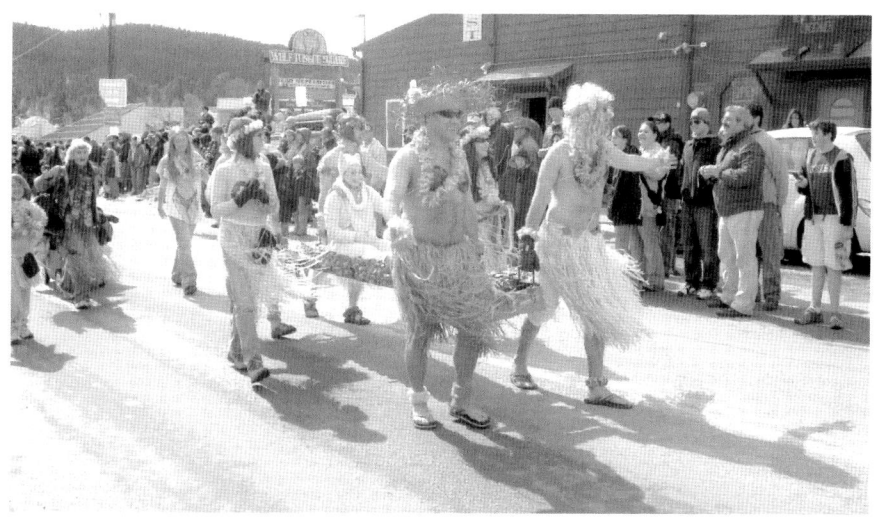

Grass skirts are nice if it doesn't snow, FDGD 2008.

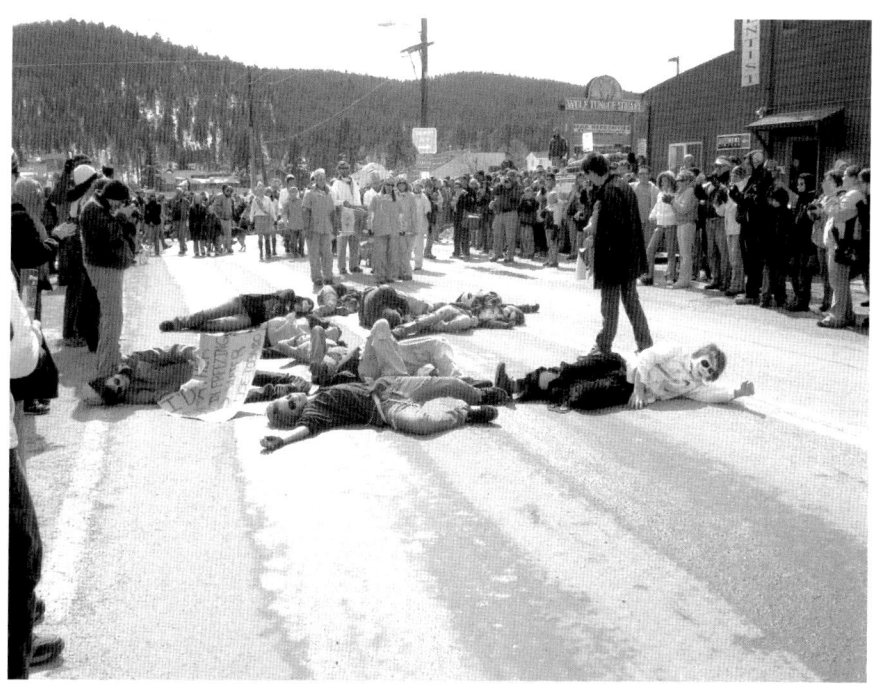

Parade zombies doing their routine, FDGD 2008.

SUVs transported them to the information center, where I met them and took them up to the shed. Everybody was as impressed with our facility as I was with a guy who thought nothing of taking a copter up the canyon for a couple hours to party. We had a great time at the shed, toasting Grandpa and telling stories.

In 2009, we had another foreign journalist following the event. Max Andrews, reporter for *Loaded* magazine in the United Kingdom and a fellow Scotsman, came over to cover the festival. *Loaded* is sort of like *Playboy*, but with the less stringent pornography laws in the EU, it comes across more like *Penthouse*. They definitely have some beautiful women in the EU. Max and I became pretty good friends over the three days, and the picture of him holding on to a rope in the back of my truck while we caromed up the road on the Midnight Champagne Tour is priceless—almost as priceless as the photo of him doing the Polar Plunge in an old-fashioned men's bathing suit, the kind that covers from wrist to ankle and goes with a handlebar moustache and a straw boater...which Max also had. With his accent and manly physique, the ladies were hanging all over him. It was hilarious, but he was digging it.

The Blue Ball was at the Black Forest again, and Halden Wolford and the High Beams Rocky Mountain Honky Tonk Band served as the musical attraction. Great music. Good dancing. The Ice Queen Contest looked more like a snow queen contest—all of the contestants were in white. It was a little weird. I took Max and a half dozen folks up to the shed for the Midnight Champagne Tour, and besides Max trying to truck ski, we had a lady who was one of those types who appears to be crazy but she's so nice that everybody just leaves her be. She brought a special dead flower to put on Bredo's box. We had a lot of fun toasting Grandpa in as many languages as we could.

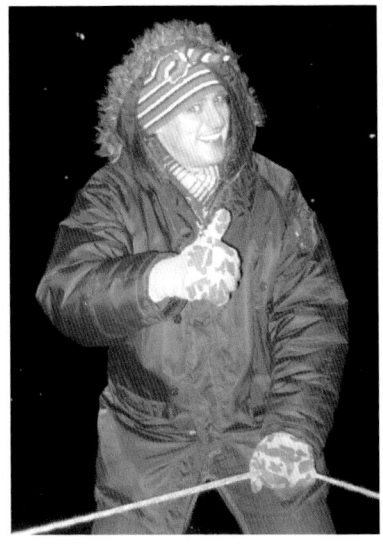

Max Andrews, reporter for the English magazine *Loaded*, taking a wild ride on the back of my truck to the 2009 Midnight Champagne Tour.

THE LATER YEARS

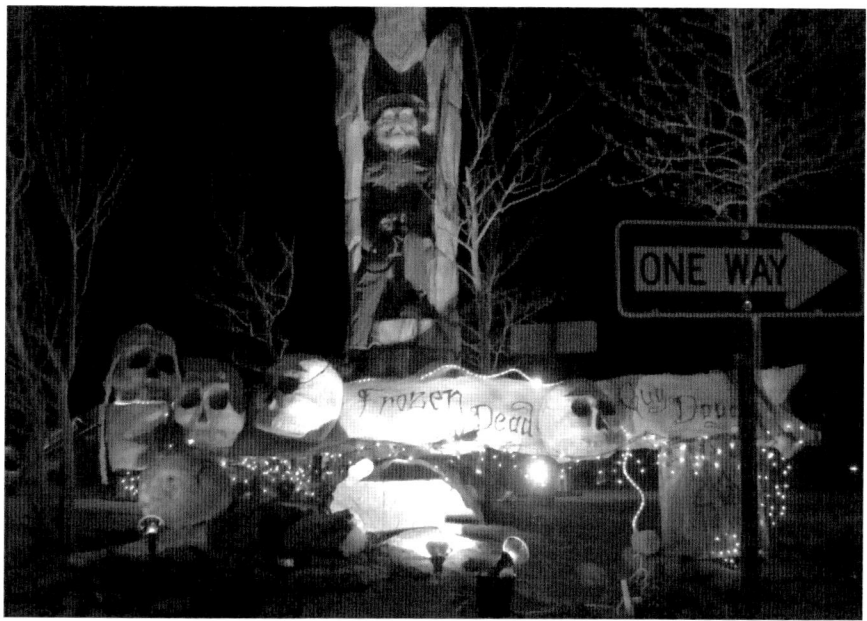

A roundabout sculpture for the 2009 FDGD.

I felt there was a subtle paradigm shift in the focus and energy of the festival this year, mostly due to the mascot. For the first time, instead of the bearded old guy, the mascot for the festival was a skull in a ski cap. To me, it went from an emphasis on an old frozen grandpa who might still be alive to a dead skull and all of the popular connotations. From life to death. Granted, it has always been about both, and always will be, but the change of emphasis was what bothered me.

In 2010, the big event this year was the reanimated tours. Trygve had finally relented and realized that the tours were good publicity and that he was missing out on the bandwagon by not allowing them. Because we were having official tours for the first time in four years, we went all out. We went around and got Gebhardt Motors, the local Beemer and Porsche dealer, to sponsor us a couple of BMW luxury SUVs and even a Porsche SUV. I didn't even know that Porsche made an SUV. They were classy, and our drivers were completely stoked, because in order to get these vehicles, they were treated like a rental. Each driver had to be responsible for and drive his car all weekend. One of my drivers who lived more than an hour's drive from

Nederland, and was going to stay in Ned at poor accommodations, ended up driving back and forth because it was so nice. He put over five hundred miles on the damn car that weekend! He was surely stylin' though.

The ball was spectacular, as Vince and Great American Taxi were back. I hung out with the band, and I even got to blow a little harp with them at one point. It was cool! In fact, we had so much fun that Vince and the band decided to take the Midnight Champagne Tour. You really ought to see the website for a proper appreciation of what happened up there that night. Suffice it to say, Vince got a little closer to communing with Grandpa than most of us (including me) ever will. I ain't gonna put my tongue on that.

The parade the next morning had great weather and was pretty long. There was a big music presence again this year, perhaps due to the big roundabout sculpture that had been in preparation for months.

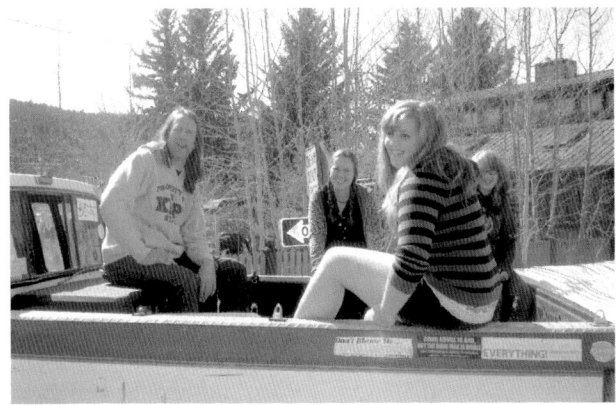

Left: Uncle Nasty, KBPI radio personality, riding in the Iceman's truck with Bo's daughter and friends in the 2010 FDGD parade.

Below: Zach's Exterminator Hearse.

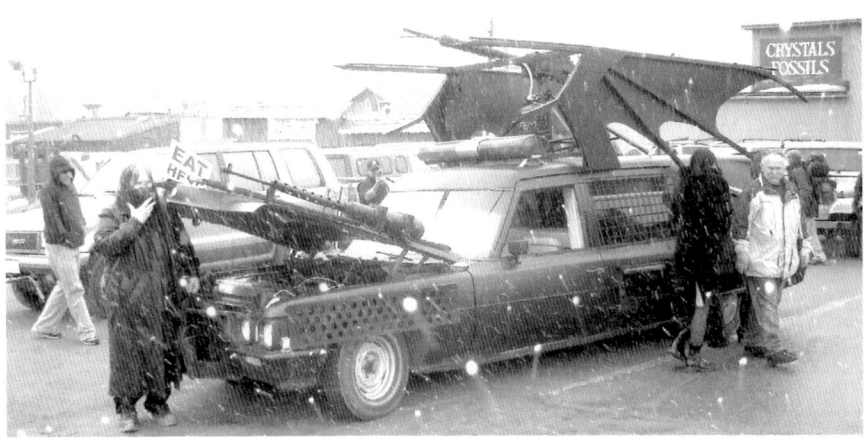

THE LATER YEARS

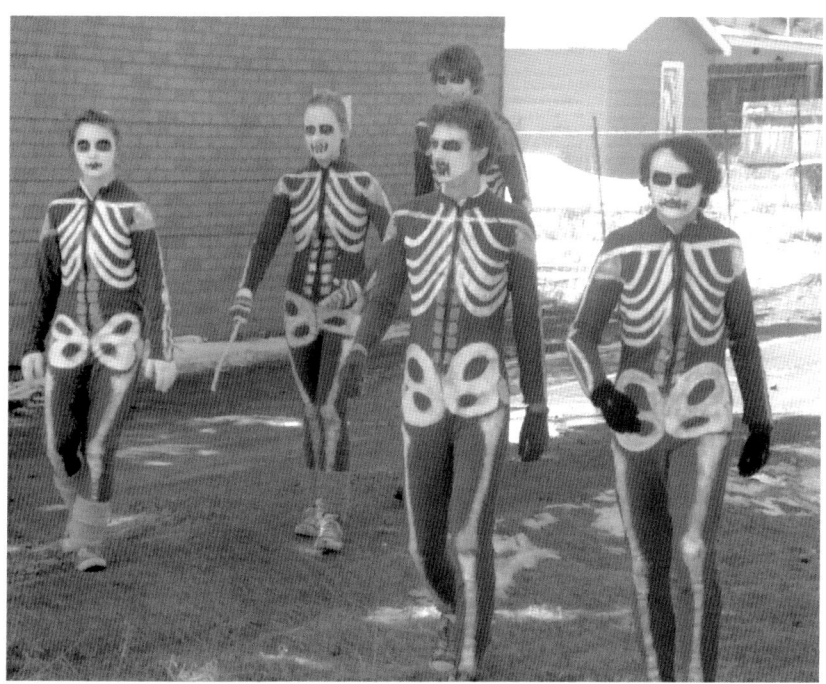

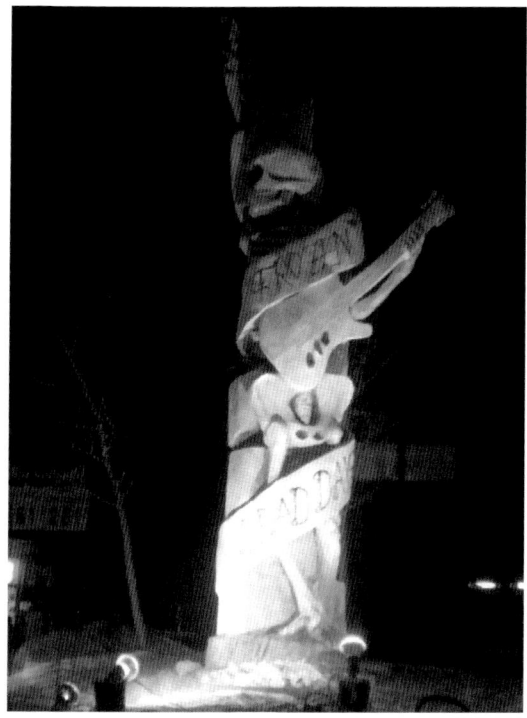

Above: The 2010 FDGD skeleton dancers.

Left: A roundabout sculpture for the 2010 FDGD.

Colorado's Iceman

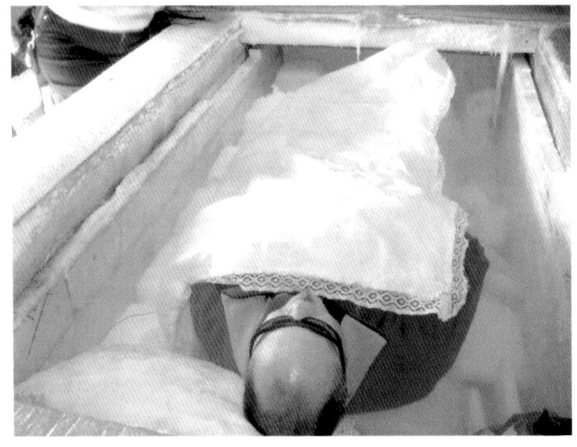

One of the tourists trying to see what it feels like. He lasted about forty-five seconds.

A twenty-foot-high, carved wooden skeleton growing out of a tree trunk that you swore could have come off a Grateful Dead album cover. In fact, there were rumors that the Dead might just stop by, as they were playing a concert that week less than one hundred miles away. That would have been totally sweet, but alas, it was just a rumor. The marshal of the parade was Uncle Nasty, a well-known DJ and personality on KBPI Rocks the Rockies, one of Denver's biggest rock radio stations. I had known Nasty for years. He was a libertarian, and we had met a couple times at various libertarian functions. In fact, I had helped steer the chamber toward making him the marshal. They needed a float for him, so naturally he got to ride in the Iceman's truck. My daughter was up for the parade that year with a couple of her friends, and she made beaucoup street cred for getting them all to ride in the back of the truck with Uncle Nasty. I did pretty well in the "you are totally amazing dad" category myself. We followed Zach's Exterminator Hearse with the batwings and flamethrowers. The skeleton dancers were behind. It was impressive.

The regular tours, due to being the first in four years, had the added attraction that you could throw some dry ice right on top of Grandpa and get your picture taken while doing it. I had brought up two giant freezers with one thousand pounds of ice, and all of the tourists got a real charge out of actually putting the ice in the chamber. I felt a little like Tom Sawyer with the whitewash. It was great getting all of these people to do my work. We had one guy who wanted to get right in and have some dry ice put on top. He did, and everyone got a great picture. We had some very fine-looking young ladies come up and pose in some very provocative ways with dry ice and Grandpa. You won't be seeing those on the website.

TOM GREEN, THE ICE HOLE AND THE GREAT LENO NO-SHOW

For three days after death, hair and fingernails continue to grow but phone calls taper off.
—*Johnny Carson*

One day I got a call from a producer who was coming to Colorado to do a segment for a show. Apparently, there was a regular segment on *The Tonight Show with Jay Leno*, with guest contributor Tom Green, that went from state to state looking for the most interesting person in each one. They would video them and then, on the show, pick a winner for the title of that state's "Most Interesting Person." They had done several states already, and it was doing well as a segment, so they were shooting five more states, and Colorado was one of them. The producer had heard of the frozen dead guy and thought that it might make a good piece. They had been to one of the ski resorts and filmed a guy who knitted ski suits, and they filmed him having his entire handmade suit unravel by tying the end of the yarn to a car and driving it across town. Not one of the better segments.

Tom Green had a way of picking up on words and making them punny. On the way out of the mountains, Tom and his crew passed a couple of guys fishing out on the lake below Georgetown. The lake runs right along the freeway there, and when Tom saw them fishing on an ice hole, he had to go over and check it out. He made a big deal out of wanting to stick his head up an "icehole," and to his credit, he actually stuck his whole head right into the icy water of the hole and came up screaming. He berated himself for actually doing it and then talked himself into doing it again. It was a pretty funny bit, Tom Green with his head in an ice hole, coming up and spewing water and screaming—not something you forget easily.

Then there was Avi, the avalanche dog. He worked at a ski resort and was a pretty good-looking mutt that had a penchant for pulling dead skiers out of snowdrifts and avalanches. He saved a guy's life once, too. Great story, nice doggy. Little did I know what part dead guys, ice and avalanches would play in the coming weeks. Now, Tom Green had done all of the other people's bits already and had saved ours for last, although it was mostly because we were on the way back to Denver and the airport. We met him and his crew in Nederland and headed up the mountain to the facility. When he got inside the shed, Tom was fascinated with the whole process of getting in and out of the cryonic chamber. When he asked Grandpa's name, he had a hard time with getting "Bredo" to come out and sound right until he hit on calling him a "Frozen Burrrredo."

Tom had a blast with that term and kept repeating it over and over until even the sound man was starting to groan every time he said it. Finally, I inadvertently slowed it down quite a bit when I tried to make a funny about having frozen nuts and how two in the box were better than one in the bag. This was a reference to the fact that Tom had had testicular cancer and had one of his testicles removed. It was well known in the comedy biz, as several comedians had made jokes about him and the issue, and I thought it might be funny with all of us guys there. However, Tom was a bit sensitive about it and took some offense. I apologized, of course, but the damage was done. Later on, the cameraman told me that while everyone made jokes about it behind his back, no one mentioned anything remotely like it to Tom's face. Oh, well…live and learn. Tom wasn't upset for long.

By the time we got everything wrapped up and all the final takes done, he was back to cracking jokes and being his own sweet self. As we were getting back into the cars, the producer walked over with Tom and said to me, "Hands down, you're the most interesting person we've seen in this entire bit, let alone in Colorado." He said that the Leno show people would have the final say but that I could probably expect a call within the next couple of weeks, as they would usually bring the winner of each state onto the show with Jay and Tom for the live bit. I was up for that. It was getting to be almost fun, having the attention focused on the cryonic preservation and the technical obstacles of this operation instead of on the wingnuts and the absurdity of it all.

Sure enough, a couple weeks later I got the call from a Leno producer, and they made all the arrangements. They flew me to Hollywood, got me in a limo from John Wayne Airport to the Universal Hilton right next to Universal Studios, wined and dined me and checked to see that I was having a good time. They flew me in on a Tuesday morning for a Wednesday taping and were flying me back Thursday afternoon. As soon as I got to the hotel, I had a sweet young intern who ran me around all the red tape and got me anything I needed. After settling in and having a bit of a late lunch (on Leno), I got a call from the producer again. The day I flew out, I saw in the papers a small story about how a guy was killed in an avalanche at one of the western Colorado ski resorts. That doesn't happen all that often, but I thought nothing of it.

Well, apparently the producers thought it was a bit in bad taste to air a segment about a dog who digs bodies out of snowdrifts the day after a guy dies in one. Remember Avi the dog? Turned out the victim was from almost the same place in Colorado. I thought it unusually sensitive for these Hollywood types, who seem to have absolutely no shame or moral character to care about offending a couple people in Hicksville, but I had to admit there was a point there. So, since I was there and the round-trip tickets were already a done deal and there wasn't much anybody could do about it, I decided to visit an old friend in San Luis Obispo and take a three-day vacation on Jay Leno's dime.

I had a great time for three days and then flew back to Colorado to await the next time they would be showing that bit, supposedly in a month. About a week later, I get a call from the Leno producer again, telling me that the next month was already overscheduled and that they had to air the segment that week. We made plans to fly out again in a couple days and got everything put on hold in my life again, anticipating another vacation to California. The morning of the day I was due to fly out, I got another call from the producer. Just that weekend, the papers had reported that Johnny Carson, Carnak the Magnificent, the longest-running and most beloved of all the hosts of the *Tonight Show*—now hosted by Jay Leno, his protégé—had died. Even I had to admit that this time, it really would be in bad taste to go on the show with Jay and offer him a Dead Guy hat…just days after Carson had died. Ouch! The producer was scrambling to get one of the other bits on as winner and eventually reached the ski patrol in Breckenridge within hours of the show and got their "man" (or dog).

So, that's how the most interesting person in Colorado turned out to be a dog named Avi, who picked dead people out of avalanches, while avalanches and dead guys bumped a frozen dead guy…and then a real dead guy bumped the frozen one and then it just all got crazy. The entire episode was full of strange coincidences, even to the point of my room number being the same as my birthday. But then that's sort of to be expected when you deal with the dead, or the undead. I'm wondering what will happen when someday I get invited back on Leno—now that he's back, too. I guess we'll just have to write that chapter when it happens.

NOTES ON NED AND THE SHED

*Life is a goddamned, stinking, treacherous game and
999 out of a thousand men are bastards.*
—*Theodore Dreiser*

One day during the festival, an incident occurred that gave me a bad taste in my mouth for the Nederland police. The previous month, I had been up to clean the place up and get it ready for the upcoming festivities. I had built a small fire in the piece of crap that passes for a wood stove in the place. It was hard to believe that they kept the place warm with that tiny, hard-to-feed, obnoxious wood stove. You'd think that Norwegians would know better. Have an airtight Jotl or something. Nope. They had this off-brand stove with half the space for wood taken up with the smoke box on top and two loosely screwed-on air vents that didn't quite shut down completely and were placed in a poor position to get a good flow and bank. So, when I made the fire and tried to damp it down, the place filled with smoke. I opened the sliding door a crack to get some air and then went about the rest of my cleaning. By the time I was ready to leave, I had completely forgotten the slightly opened door, and it really wasn't very visible anyway. I missed it in my final sweep and headed on back down the hill, leaving the sliding door ever so slightly open.

Of course, three weeks later, when I went back up right before the festival, I remembered it. When I went to close it, I noticed that it was already closed but not locked. Odd. On my way out of town, I stopped by the police station and had a word with the chief, Ken Robinson. Now, the police in Ned have undergone several changes since I've been going there. Long gone are the days when an illegal alien could be on the force, even if he was a fellow highlander. "Scotty" was a good cop, though, and the Ned police force was poorer without him. Well, after a couple years of struggling with who was really in charge, Nederland or the Sheriff's Department, they had finally settled on their own police chief with their own couple of police guys. I had run afoul of them recently when I had allegedly run a stop sign. When the cop caught up to me, on the other side of town, I was not too happy about it. Ken had interceded at that time, hearing who I was on the radio, and they let me go with a warning. I was miffed at the (somewhat) trumped-up charge but was thankful for the courtesy. So I felt pretty friendly toward the chief; he seemed like a reasonable guy, and he apparently liked me. When I walked in and sat down in his office, I told him about the door. He said that he had been sending patrols up there to keep an eye on the place with the festival approaching and all, but no one had reported anything. He wasn't really all that concerned, as there was just a door that may or may not have been left open and there wasn't really much he could do anyway. I left feeling not quite right.

The next weekend at the festival, I wrapped up the last tour of the morning and was headed down to the parade; I was not due back at the facility until after noon. I had radioed to the base station that I was leaving, and then I took a little break before I jumped back into my truck and headed back into town. So, it was about fifteen minutes later than I had anticipated that I was driving down the little road onto which the property driveway dumps. When I hit the main road out of the subdivision (a slightly less rutted dirt road), I ran into a cop turning onto the little road. We stopped and I chatted a minute with him, asking what was up. He said that he had a couple of people who were looking for a friend who was lost. I told him that I had just come from the shed and that there was no one around there that I saw. He said thanks, and we both drove off in opposite directions. Mountain roads have an interesting habit of switching back and forth to get down steep hills. I was just starting to make the last switchback, after which I wouldn't be able to see the property, when I caught a glimpse in my mirror of the cop car headed straight into the property's driveway instead of switching back to visit the neighbors up the road, like he said he was going to.

Being suspicious is part of my nature. I also have a weird habit of sometimes being in the right place at the right time. I was once hiking with a fellow Eagle Scout and my soon-to-be wife in the canyon above Boulder Falls. My friend and I had just eased our height-challenged young lady down from a rather steep cliff face and were being (somewhat) playfully battered about the head and shoulders for being so damn stupid as to take her to her worst nightmare (of being thrown off a cliff). "Eagle Scouts ought to know better than that!" she was saying to us over and over as we were walking down the creek—and not over that damn ridge again. So, when we came to a group of people gathered around a log over the creek, we were more than glad to stop for a minute and offer our point of view.

Some people had gotten across the creek upstream earlier and now were trying to get back across right above the falls. There was a small log jammed in the rocks that spanned the creek at about water level. Everybody had gotten back across except for one rather hefty girl, who was balking at walking across the log and was going to shimmy along it on her ample butt instead. Having just used our rope to save the young damsel from her rocky tower, my friend and I suggested that perhaps these folks might find it prudent to fasten the rope around their friend, just in case. Be prepared—that's the Eagle Scout motto. So we showed them how to tie a secure knot (bowline, of course), and they tossed the rope over to the girl, who secured it around herself and started to slide along the log. About halfway across, where the water was pretty deep and moving fastest, she slipped and went under the log and headed right for the falls. Fortunately, the rope held, and even though it was touch and go for a second or two, we all pulled like hell and dragged her back from under the log and out on the shore. She was shaking like a leaf, especially since that year two other people had already gone over the falls and died. Just another good deed per day in the life of an Eagle Scout.

And then there was the time at the Stones concert in Boulder when I saved a female friend from a crowd of toughs by threatening them from above, where they couldn't reach me. I didn't even know that my best friend's girl was at the concert, and I found myself in the unique position to help her out of a potentially bad situation when no one else was around. And then there was another time…but you get the picture. I have a knack of acting on impulses, and they turn out to have far-reaching implications. So seeing the cop car go straight when it should have turned back made me turn right around and head back to the property myself.

When I pulled up, I saw the cop car parked in front of me. As I stopped and got out of my truck, a couple of people ran from around the back of the building (where the aforementioned unlocked door was) and jumped straight back into the cop car as the cop himself walked on by and approached me. At first, he was all blustery and pulling his rank as a cop. He said that they were just looking for someone. Being well versed in these things, I nailed him with trespassing unless he had a warrant. He tried to bull his way over me, but I just started to jump all over his case—just what the hell was going on here. He changed his story from looking for a suspect to looking for a lost friend to looking for a drunk friend to, finally, just looking. I was still verbally beating his ass, though I was thinking of cutting him some slack since there was no harm done, when he started to change his tune and suck up to me. He started babbling about how he had voted for me for sheriff and how great a guy I was; then I really started to smell a rat. I told him to get in his car and get off the property and that I'd just forget this ever happened.

I went back around the place and saw where they had walked up to the door that was supposed to be unlocked almost immediately when they got out of the car—just in the few minutes it took me to turn around and drive back up there. It's like they knew that the door was unlocked. I decided to take a good look around, mostly for evidence that someone had been inside. In the process of evaluating the interior, I noticed that a painting, an original watercolor signed by Bredo himself, was not with the other paintings. I couldn't say when that painting had disappeared, but it sure wasn't there now. I looked high and low for it. It wasn't anywhere. It was an illustration that Bredo had done of an old Norwegian fairy tale. It was an image of a man in a black outfit and cap, carrying a child and jumping over a narrow but deep chasm with woods on both sides. It was kind of a tall, thin painting. Nothing else was missing as far as I could tell. I hadn't seen anything in the hands of the people with the cop, but they really hadn't had time to go inside anyway. I started to think that it wasn't the cop's first visit to the place and wondered just how many people he had brought by in those weeks when the door was unlocked—and no one reported it to me.

I went down the hill finally and went to the sheriff's office. When I told the chief about what had happened, he sort of pooh-poohed the idea that any of his officers would be doing anything like that and said that he'd look into it. I wasn't impressed. A few weeks later, when I was up in Ned again, I stopped in and asked him what he had found out. He said that his officer was looking for someone and hadn't called it in but that it was on the report (filed after the fact) and that everything seemed fine. He said that his guys would never do anything unseemly. Yeah, I thought to myself, that's why he tried to weasel out and sweet-talk me up there that day. He's an honest and upright cop. Right.

Notes on Ned and the Shed

Since Ken wasn't going to give me any satisfaction, I decided to do a little investigating on my own. I have some influence in the law enforcement community, having run for sheriff and trained with sheriff's deputies and even been on the shooting range with them from time to time. They all know me as a staunch libertarian and an advocate for personal responsibility. I put out a couple of feelers and inquiries about the law enforcement history of the Ned deputy and where he had been in Boulder County. When my contacts got back to me, the story they told was pretty weird, but it all made sense.

This guy was a former Boulder City cop and was on the force back when JonBenét Ramsey was killed. In fact, he was involved in the investigation itself and got tangled up in a scheme to sell crime scene photos to the media, along with another officer, a few weeks after the murder. It was all kept pretty quiet, as there were both sheriff personnel and city police personnel involved. The upshot of it was, this guy was quietly reprimanded and kicked off the city force, and then he turned up at the Sheriff's Department a little later, where he got involved with searching fellow officers' lockers at work and eventually was let go from the Sheriff's Department for that incident. Again, it was kept on the QT, as no one likes to hear about a bad cop. This was all in the preceding five to six years, and now this guy had turned up on the Ned police force, where the chief was defending him on charges of furthering his own gain with celebrity theft? When he has a history of it? Unfortunately, as all of my information was unofficial, there wasn't much I could do about anything. I just kept a weather eye out for any Ned police poking around and watched myself closely to ensure no more mistakes. I did notice that the guy was released from the Ned police force after a few months and eventually turned up as police chief in Lochbuie, a small Colorado plains community where they probably never heard of JonBenét or the frozen dead guy. But I've got my feelers out. I know people in Lochbuie. I've told them to be on the lookout for that peculiar painting. I'll find it someday.

There are bad guys and there are good guys. Some of the good guys are the ice guys. Ice guys make up the elite group who have assisted me over the years to carry ice up to Grandpa, and they sometimes help out at the festivals. I started out using the guys who worked for me at DTI. But the highly skilled and expensive labor from Delta was not economically feasible when we were on a shoestring budget anyway, so I soon found another, cheaper source of labor at my dear ol' alma mater, CU. The university runs a "help wanted" electronic bulletin board, and I ran an ongoing ad there for many years: "Ice

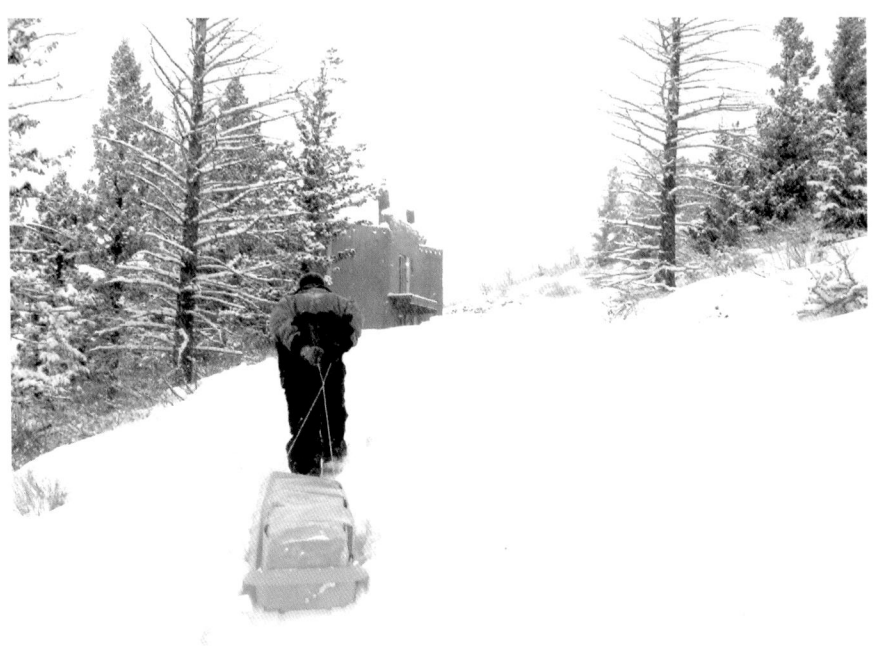

Hauling the ice on sleds up the last portion of the road.

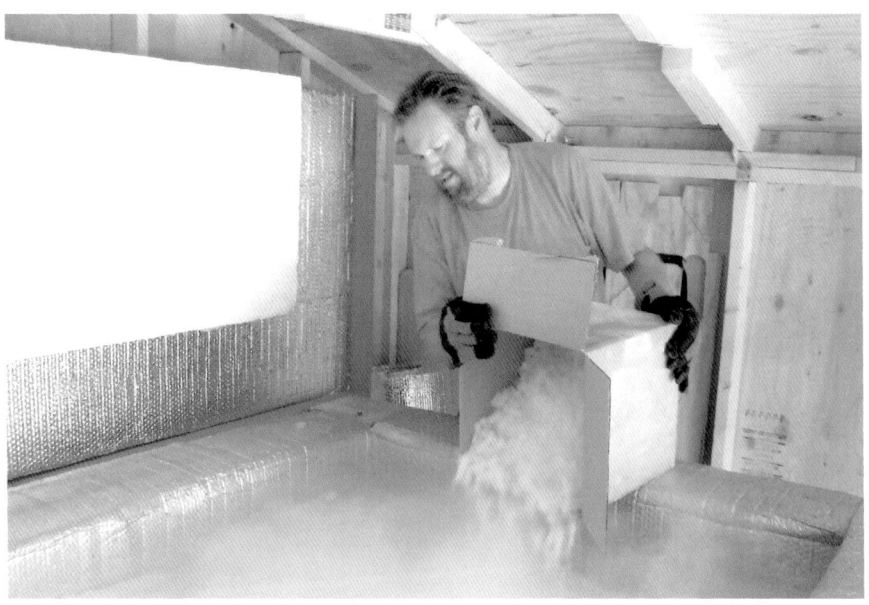

Gary the assistant dumping in dry ice pellets.

Labor needed. Ability to lift 100 pounds and tolerance for cold and dead bodies a must." I got a lot of calls at the beginning of each semester, and I would put all of the applicants who passed the requirements onto an e-mail list. Every month I would query the list as to who was available and who wasn't. The college kids were perfect for a once-a-month job that only paid twenty-five dollars and lunch, but it looked great on a résumé and gave them something to talk about to their friends.

The résumé thing was serious. I had an ice guy come back to me several years after he had graduated, and he told me that being an ice guy got him his job. Apparently the job selection was down to my ice guy and one other. They both had almost identical résumés, went to the same school and everything. When the prospective employer saw the FDG Ice Delivery Guy on his résumé, he started to get excited and asked a lot of questions. He was a fan and really was impressed that my guy had not only delivered ice there but also actually had a picture of it posted on the web with him standing next to Grandpa's cryonic chamber. My ice guy got the job.

Ice guys have also been friends and neighbors. In the early years, an old friend, Dave W., would go along, and we'd think of ways to promote the dead guy. He really had the idea to make a frozen dead guy documentary first. The trouble was that he wasn't much of a videographer. He'd forget to turn off the video cam and ended up with half a tape of his leg in the car. He also had a bad habit of cutting off your head. He'd get so involved in directing that he'd forget he was trying to hold the camera on something and end up videotaping the ground. The footage he ended up with is pretty hilarious but not too marketable.

I've had the sons of old next-door neighbors look me up years after they moved and ask to do an ice run. I've had sons and fathers go along for a special birthday treat. Sometimes, I even had special events and announced them in an e-mail that I sent to a select list of "FDG Interest" people (over the years they had asked me to keep them informed about what's going on). Even my dog, Gillian, would get into the act. She loved to climb up, sit on the top of Grandpa's chamber and chew on pieces of frost that collected on dropped dry ice pieces. She was also the best danged watchdog there ever was—Gillian the Fat Wonder Dog.

Sometimes me and the ice guys would get a little bored, and so we'd sit around and talk to Grandpa like he was listening. He's a great listener. We'd sometimes see images of him in our minds like he might be if he were a ghost or something. Breathing in too much carbon dioxide does funny things to a man!

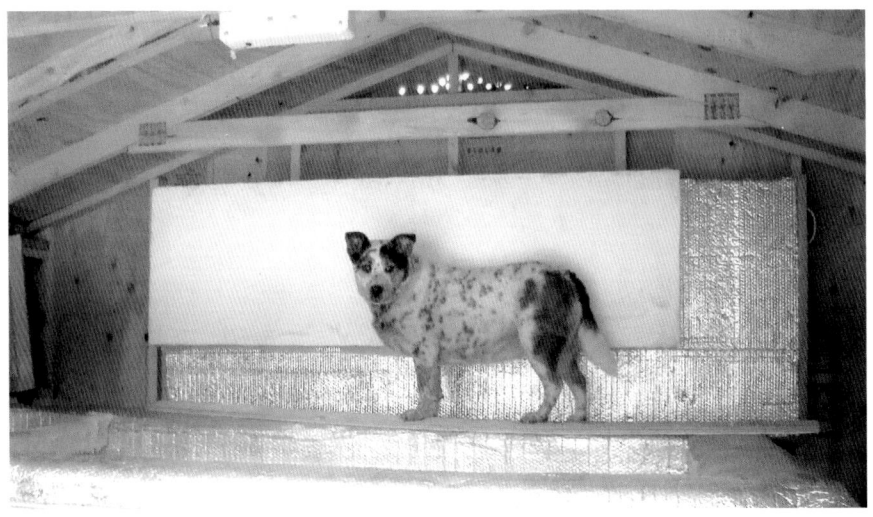

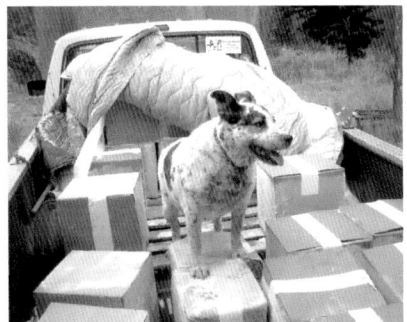
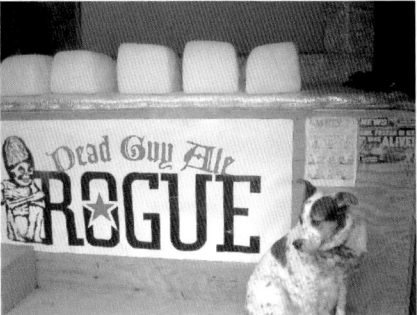

Gillian guarding the cryonic chamber and the dry ice.

Sometimes being the Iceman or an ice guy is damn hard work. It may look pretty, but when the weather gets ornery it can be pretty ugly. We've delivered in rain, snow, sun, dead of night—the ice must get through! Over the years, there have been several times when either the four-wheel drive failed or there was just too much drifted snow, and all of the ice had to be transported in sleds or just plain carried by hand the last hundred yards or so, uphill, usually in a blizzard. That's a tale that grows with the telling and will be told to great-grandchildren sitting on knees.

We have used blocks, slabs, pellets and rice forms of dry ice. Sometimes it depended on the supply. During the Dry Ice Wars, the outfit we used had its own $250,000 machine that spit out a sixty-pound block every seven

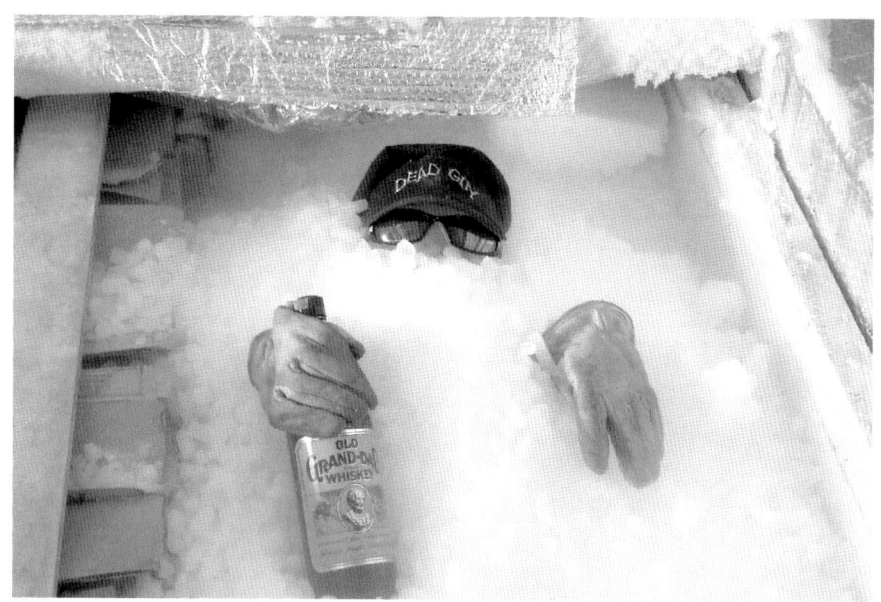

Getting silly with Grandpa on dry ice.

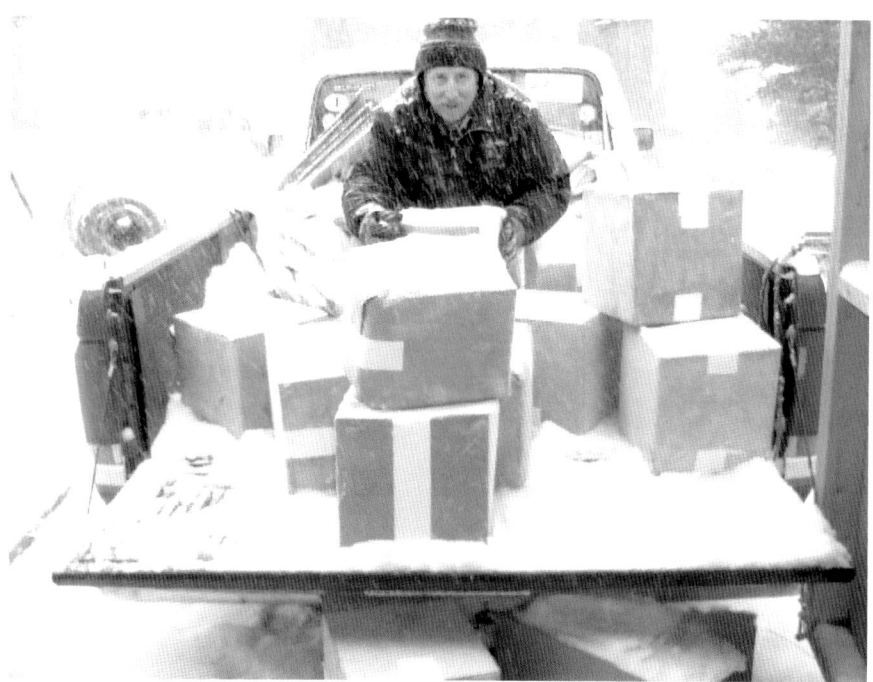

Bo unloading ice in a snowstorm.

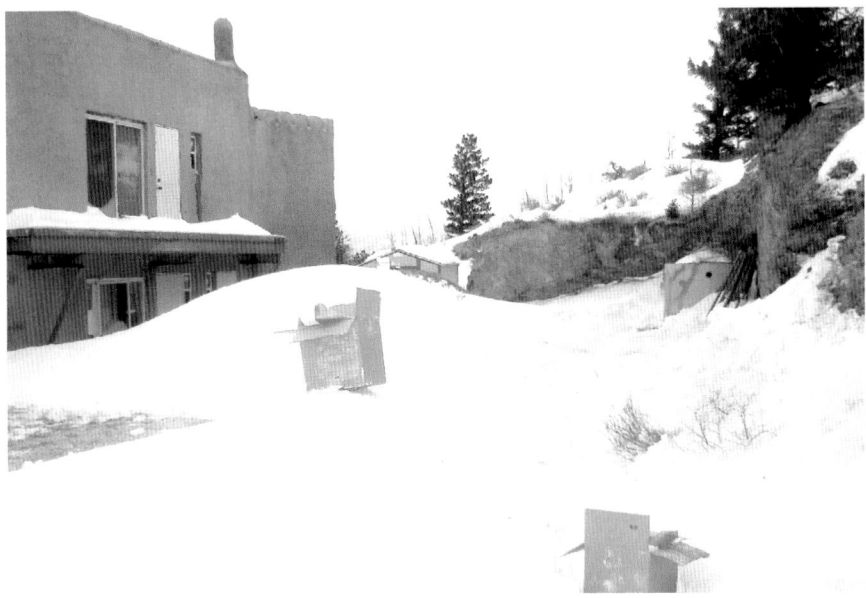

Hand-carrying fifty-pound boxes of dry ice to the snowed-in shed.

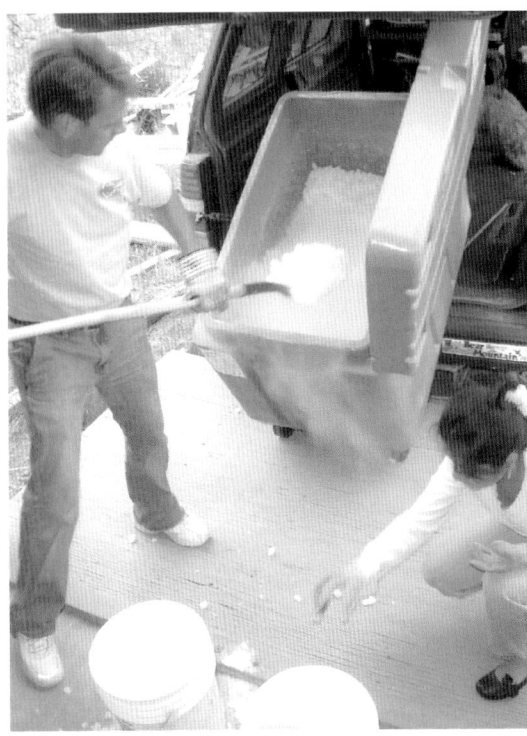

Ice guys shoveling dry ice pellets.

minutes. We used blocks exclusively while we were with that company. Later, we had a supplier that had pellets. Now, pellets of dry ice make things very cold very fast but sublimate quickly. Blocks maintain cold temperatures longer, being a solid mass, but take a while to cool things down, due to minimal contact. We used both for a while, one for cold power and one for staying power. We'd transport boxes of pellets, or sometimes an entire cooler full, and either pour 'em in or shovel 'em in.

Sometimes the job requires an iron will and serious cojones—like when I jumped in at the Polar Bear New Year's Day Polar Plunge. Trygve had founded the Boulder Polar Bear Club back in 1984, and when the twentieth anniversary plunge was scheduled, I decided to do a memorial plunge and wear the T-shirt that Trygve made for himself as founder of the club. I actually am a fond believer in ice plunging…but only after sitting in a hot tub for an hour or so. I do not like it the other way around. But I took one for the Gipper and did a publicity thing, and I was really glad that it was a nice day that year.

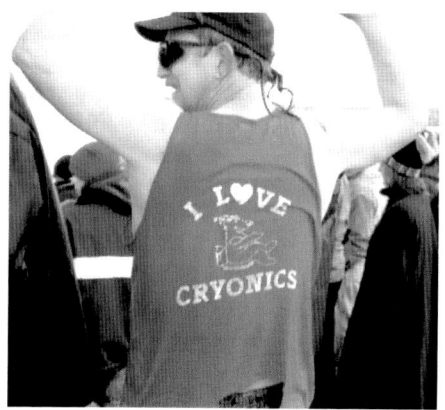

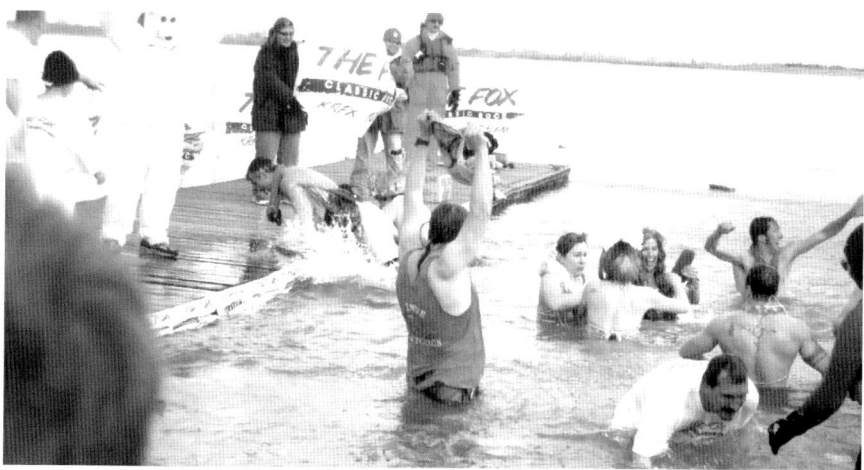

Top: Bo taking the New Year's Day Polar Bear Club twentieth anniversary Polar Plunge with founder Trygve Bauge's original cryonics polar bear T-shirt.

Bottom: Bo, wearing the founder's T-shirt at the twentieth anniversary Polar Bear Club Polar Plunge.

Sometimes, it takes outside teamwork to make it happen. I've had truck trouble and have gotten the mechanic to squeeze me in so I can still make the run in time. I have a backup plan that involves renting a flatbed from Home Depot if I ever break down so far that I have to transfer the ice. I've been sick, and the doc takes me in between patients to get me fixed up enough to do the run. Doc Blaich also takes care of me when I lift the ice too many times. There are runs where we lift each block four times. That's six thousand pounds, or three tons. A good kinesiologist really can help. A great one works wonders. It's really funny how so many people are fascinated by this and are willing to help out. I guess everyone sort of feels sorry for Bredo and wants to do what they can for a guy who can't really do much on his own.

PSYCHIC PHENOM

When we have shuffled off this mortal coil…
—William Shakespeare

Over the years, I've had several groups of psychics come up to the shed to try and determine what, if anything, Grandpa thinks about all of this. My initial concern was that in my day-to-day activities, I tend to piss off people quite regularly, and sometimes it's not so good. What if I was upsetting this dead guy's plans or something by preserving his earthly remains and preventing him from going to wherever it is people go when they die? What if he was about ready to haunt those responsible? It's not like I had a lot of experience in dealing with dead people or anything, but I had been doing the job for several years. One day, when I read in the paper about a group in Boulder called the Boulder Psychic Institute (BPI), I thought to myself, "Now, there's an outfit that might be interested in doing some research on a dead guy." So, I contacted the company and had a little chat.

I talked with the head of the organization, a guy named Michael, and we arranged to have a teaching and research session at the shed. He would bring his top psychic (himself) and his assistant (his wife), as well as a couple of promising students, up to the shed and do a series of séances, with us filming and documenting the procedure. I would work up a series of questions and would ask each psychic certain ones that I would reword and ask the other psychics, too. I intended to compare responses and see if there was any regularity to the answers—or find out if they were just pulling it out of their asses.

Taking my cues from Houdini, I tried to remove any collaboration or signaling opportunities by keeping each psychic isolated from the others until after all of them were given the opportunity to perform. I had each of the psychics ask the same questions of Grandpa and hoped to be able to compare responses. We even tossed in a question that nobody knew, just to see how consistent the answers would be: "Which direction is his head?" It was either facing to the west or to the east. We didn't know. Trygve didn't know. Nobody knew. The stainless steel sarcophagus looks the same at both ends. There are two wire leads coming out of it that are attached to tags and, I assume, to temperature sensors inside the sarcophagus itself. One tag says "Head" and the other "Ankle." The two tags come out of the same end of the sarcophagus and are about the same length. No one knows which is heads and which is tails.

When a cryonically preserved body is kept at a high-tech facility, they keep it in liquid nitrogen, a standard cryogenic temperature–producing agent. They also keep the bodies in what is essentially a large thermos bottle, called a dewar. They store them upright to minimize the evaporation and, naturally, keep the body head-down to make sure the most important parts get the most cryo-preservation. They put a temperature sensor in the head and one in the foot to monitor the temperature and the LN levels. When the foot temperature starts to drop, they know that it's time for more LN, and the head stays the same temperature all the time. There are those folks who are into cryonics who don't have much money or imagination and opt for what they call a "Neuro." That's where they whack your head off and toss it into a vat of liquid nitrogen. Yum. More on cryonics later.

So, when the day came, I got my crew of psychics together, and we headed up to Nederland, where I usually meet everyone who wants to go see Grandpa. Gives 'em time to soak in the flavor of Nederland. We rendezvoused at the info booth, which strangely enough I had to give them directions to find. You'd think they'd know that. We headed up to the property, and when we got there, I sent one of my guys to keep an eye on the psychics and watch that they didn't talk to one another. The rest of us went and set up the video camera in the shed and got ready to record the session with each psychic. We brought in the head honcho, Michael, and asked him a couple of preliminary questions. Then we asked him if he could feel Grandpa's presence. He closed his eyes and started to talk to himself about what he saw, and after a few minutes of concentrating and looking like he was trying to sense something he started to chuckle. He mumbled a few things and then started to laugh. He said aside to us, "I've found his spirit, but he doesn't know he's dead." He continued to rock back and forth with his eyes closed, a little like Stevie Wonder, giving us updates every couple of minutes.

"He's skiing—in Norway…He doesn't believe me when I tell him he's dead…I'm bringing him over here to see his body…I'm showing him his body," he said.

Finally, he was able to convince Bredo that he really was dead, and we started to ask him our questions. The first and foremost question was, "Are you upset in any way by our actions?" We got back a negative. Whew! Whether or not it was true, I felt better knowing that we weren't pissing off the dead. When we asked whether he "approved" of this cryonic preservation or not, the answer was that if his grandson wanted to throw away his money on such things, who was he (Bredo) to say no. Pretty libertarian of the old guy, I thought. Then we asked him whether he himself thought that the cryonics thing was a good idea or not.

"Why would I want that old decrepit body back?" he answered, which I thought was pretty reasonable. Even after "explaining" the concept of cryonics being able to restore you to the condition you were in before you died, he seemed unconvinced and thought that we were foolish to think that he would want anything to do with his former "vessel," or "holder" as Michael translated it. Michael didn't come out with direct statements. It was more like he was getting impressions and had to translate them into words we could understand. Later, we watched the video multiple times to try to see Michael at the moment of contact.

After Michael, we took each of the other psychics into the shed, videotaped them as they got their impressions and asked them the same questions for comparisons. All in all, we collected more than four hours of tape and wanted to wait until we could get it back to the studio to analyze it and compare notes. The full report on that research is still classified in DTI archives, but suffice it to say, we were satisfied that we weren't making any spiritual waves with what we heard. It was interesting that we got the most varied response to the question for which no one knew an answer. Two wests, an east and an "I can't tell." I think the latter was perhaps the most honest.

There's an epilogue to this incident—or, as Paul Harvey would put it, the "rest of the story." Several months after the visit to the shed, I wanted to get back in touch with BPI and ask a couple of follow-up questions that our analysis had produced. I called and called, but there was no response for over a week. I finally went to Boulder and dropped by the offices one afternoon. The place was closed, and it looked like nobody was around.

While investigating a little further, I ran into a guy who appeared to be looking for BPI, too. He turned out to be the owner of the building and was looking for his tenants. He said that their rent was paid up but that they had just disappeared—no forwarding addresses, no notice to move, nothing. He said that they had been good tenants for many months and was quite puzzled by their lack of communication with him. They apparently had disappeared off the face of the earth. Was Bredo pissed that Michael told him that he was dead? Food for thought.

The next set of psychics came up several years later with A. Whitney Brown on a Comedy Central spot. I thought that they were pretty self-serving and seemed to be pushing their own agenda of not being happy with the hoopla surrounding Grandpa rather than channeling Bredo himself. Those so-called psychics were pretty lame, as was another group, from the Psychic Network, that contacted me once to come and do readings on Bredo. They appeared to be strictly commercial, and the guy who led the three up there reminded me of the interior designer in *Beetlejuice*—greasy and obviously a fraud. Didn't hear from them again.

The last psychic I talked to was a bit more on the up and up. I was invited to attend a reading of a psychic mystery book that had made a brief mention of us. It was in a Boulder bookstore, and there were many people there from many walks of life. After the reading, one of the ladies approached me, and we started to chat about Grandpa. She said that she was a psychic and had followed the story of Grandpa with some amusement. In the course of our conversation, she mentioned that she used to feel his presence up there in Ned once in a while but that it seemed that he had moved on and she couldn't feel him anymore. I thought that was interesting, and we chatted further about the role of spirits in our culture and religion.

The results of these psychic experiments are difficult to interpret, but in light of my own personal philosophies and beliefs, along with what I know about the principles involved, I put forward the following explanation.

In my studies on the dead, it appears that often a spirit can be so enamored of life that it has a difficult time leaving this plane of existence. Ghosts are a good example of this. Most if not all ghosts have a deep connection with whatever they haunt: a favorite resting place, a murdered loved one, unrequited love, things like that. Grandpa Bredo had a deep love of his Norwegian woods and skiing. According to Trygve, Bredo was very disappointed that in his later years he was unable to ski like he used to. Time in the hereafter is also thought to be on a different scale than in this plane. It is therefore within the realm of possibilities that Bredo went to his beloved slopes after he died to get it out of his system, so to speak. Not knowing that he was dead, he skied like it was real, which it was for him. When the first psychic brought it to his attention that he was dead, it was possibly part of the overall plan. You have to move on some day. Whether or not Bredo was upset at the people who brought reality crashing around his spectral ears is up for debate, but their disappearance was a bit odd. However, once Bredo was informed of his state of being, he would then, by my philosophies, start to prepare for the next phase: reincarnation. Thus, a short time later, there appears to be no psychic contacts with what was "Bredo Morstoel" since he had moved on to his next lesson and life.

There is a rather large difference between the philosophies required to believe in cryonics and those for believing in reincarnation. That was one of the driving reasons for the development of the International Cryonics Institute.

ICICLE

*My grandmother's brain was dead, but her heart was still beating.
It was the first time we ever had a Democrat in the family.*
−Emo Phillips

The International Cryonics Institute and Center for Life Extension, or IC Institute as we call it, was brought about by a need for a deep understanding of the principles involved in life extension, which is the whole raison d'être for cryonics. It was also to give us some street cred.

For several years, at each festival, there would be a display from a national cryonics outfit called Cryonics Advocacy Group (CAG). It was founded by a lady by the name of Kennita Watson. She advocates education for the people and is very libertarian. I would hear things from her concerning how the "legitimate" cryonics community was afraid that we were giving cryonics a bad name. Funny stuff.

The second year she came, she brought a mysterious assistant. He looked like a fugitive from ZZ Top—long beard, ball cap and dark glasses—and he was skinny and quiet. He and I had some discussions about cryonics, but I never found out who he was. He would tell me that keeping a body on dry ice was a completely inferior way to cryonically preserve a client. I would counter that with the nanotechnology solution envisioned by most cryonicists, it wouldn't be a problem to rebuild the body no matter what the condition, as long as all of it was there. You could theoretically reanimate a mummy (if you had all the jars) or the Iceman (my namesake) they found in the glacier in Europe. It's all there; just add water…and nanobots. He didn't agree, but I could tell from the discussion that he wasn't just a tyro at cryonics. It was several years later that I was to learn that he was a big wheel in the international cryonics community and was one of the directors of the biggest "legitimate" cryonics company in America. He had worn a disguise because he didn't want to be recognized or be thought to endorse our backyard cryonics in any way, even by attending. I'll just call him M from A. M and I still have discussions by e-mail these days. After the publication of *Frozen*, however, a tell-all book about the "legitimate" cryonics business and the shenanigans with Ted Williams, he's kept a pretty low profile. But he got me thinking that year about how to make us a little more respectable.

Trygve has always been into life extension—hence the cryonic preservation, the ice bathing, the macro diet. All of the stuff that Trygve believes in and practices is meant to extend his life and improve its quality. We are certainly an international operation, with the financing coming from Norway and the operation in the United States. So I first came up with the International Cryonics Institute or "ICI," which I thought was pretty clever. Then I realized that Cryonic Life Extension Institute wasn't bad, but when I put it together with ICI and got ICICLEI, I racked my brain for a different "c" because two "cryonics" and two "institutes" in the name was straight out of the department of redundancy department. Then I hit on the International Cryonics Institute and Center for Life Extension, and ICICLE was born. It was too perfect not to use it. It perfectly described our operation and was about as catchy as you can get. Even the short version worked well—the IC Institute.

Inspired by the name, I decided to give us as much legitimacy as possible. I bought the "icinstitute" domain, and I initiated a Web page with a monthly "Ice Run Report," complete with pictures.

In the beginning, I only kept ice sales receipts and made periodic e-mail reports to Trygve. In 1999, one of my ice guy assistants donated a logbook, and we started to log every trip. That logbook is in the archives now. In 2002, I switched to all e-mail reports and just printed them out for the monthly report. In 2004, the ice log was published on the Frozen Dead Guy website (frozendeadguy.com of course). Starting in 2005, the ice log was moved to the IC Institute website and remains there to this day, testimony to the tenacity of DTI planetary ecologists.

Along with the website came classy addresses—director@icinstitute.us for example. I put it in the "us" extension, because although we're international, we're based in the United States. Besides, there are a couple of other IC Institutes in the world, and they had snatched the ".com" and ".biz" already—not to mention the fact that it distanced us a little from the Frozen Dead Guy website. I mean it is really easy to give out the web address for FDG, but it is a bit commercial for a research facility.

The Frozen Dead Guy website came to me back in 2002. When the hype started up for the FDGD festival, an Internet entrepreneur thought that he'd buy the FDG domain and make a few bucks off selling it to the festival. Who didn't try to buy a domain they thought they could sell to the right people back in those days? Well, this guy got into a bit of a struggle with the chamber over the trademark registration of the FDG name. To register a name, you have to sell something with that name on it. The chamber in Ned sells festival gear with "Frozen Dead Guy Days" on it—shirts, hats, hoodies, underwear, you name it. The chamber has a registered trademark for Frozen Dead Guy Days, and it tends to defend its trademark. The members also had no desire to pay any money for a website when they had their own already and used it to promote FDG stuff.

The guy was stuck with a domain no one wanted and faced possible litigation against him if he tried to make money off the registered name. So he called me up one day after the festival and offered me the domain free of charge. I could take over the rest of his registration and then register it in whatever name I wanted when the registration expired in a few months. He said that while he couldn't buck the chamber over the name, *I* probably could. He even tried to talk me into going after the chamber because I had first rights to the name and because the chamber probably infringed on me. I believe that he had had some harsh words with the chamber over all of this and wasn't feeling too disposed toward them. I politely declined to interfere in the relationship between the chamber and myself but said thanks for the domain and started to work out a website. It was easy to tell people the web address, and I started to fill it with the background stories from all of the newspapers and TV coverage over the years. I put links to Trygve's Meta Portal and other cryonic sites. It worked well for many years, but the IC Institute needed its own, more research-oriented website.

The research we do is a bit esoteric, but it does have value. We are one of only six cryonic storage facilities in the entire world. We are the foremost authorities on backyard, DIY-style cryonics. We do photographic crystallography studies on the crystals in the cryonic chamber. We study the long-term storage effect on perishables like cake and ice cream. Every time we throw a birthday party for Grandpa, and there have been several, we save some of the cake and ice cream to see how well it stays preserved. I've tasted ten-year-old cake saved from Bredo's 101st birthday party; while

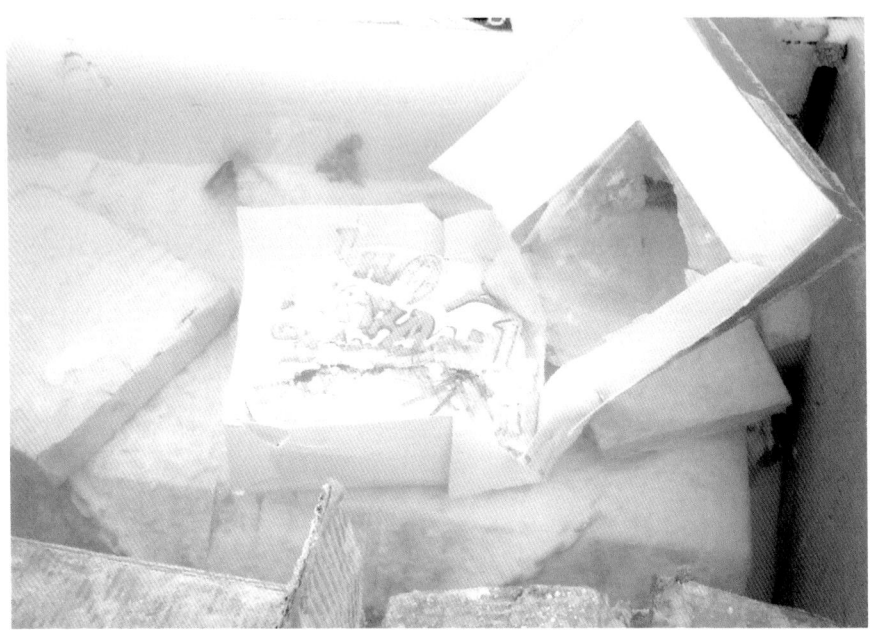

Above: Bredo's 101st birthday cake.

Below: Bo toasting Bredo on the latter's 101st birthday.

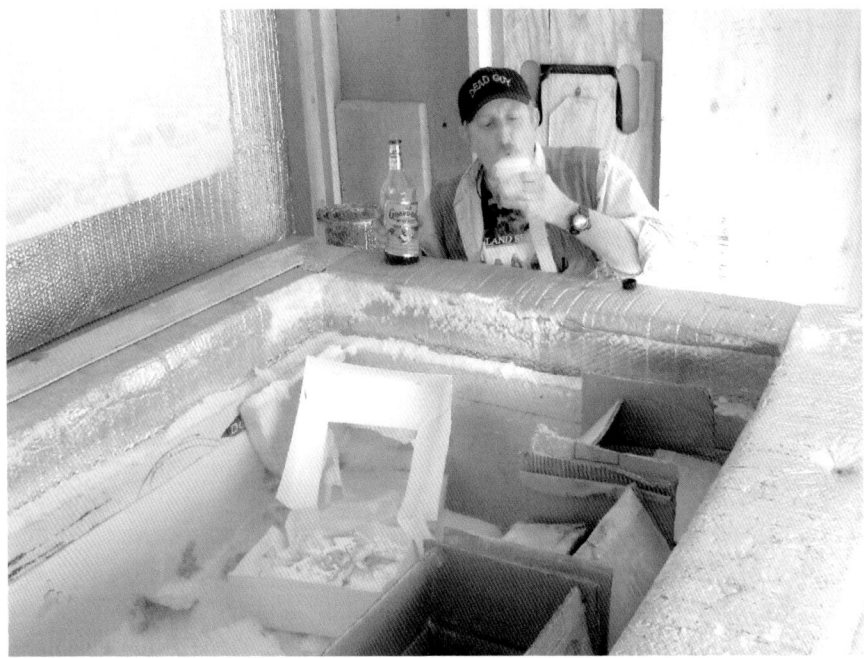

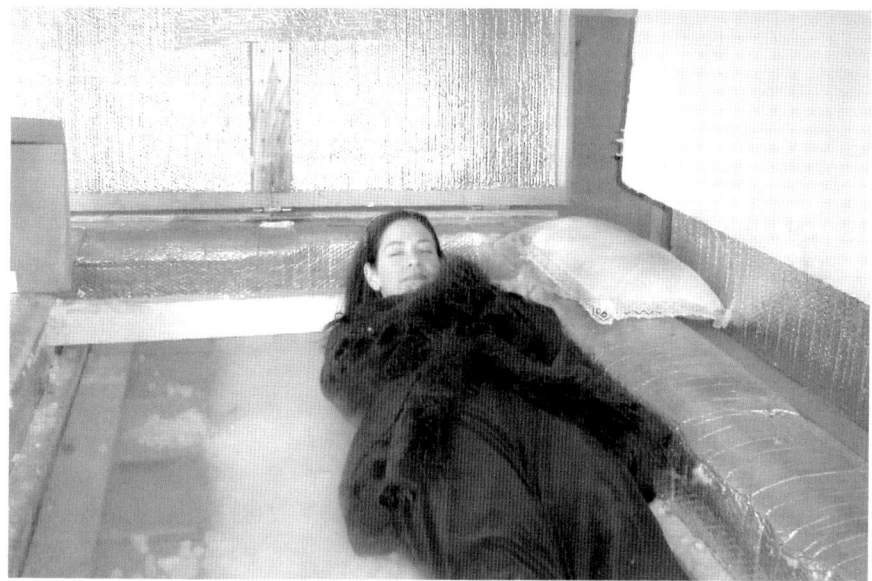

Marci checks out what it's like being Grandpa at the Grave Digger's Lunch.

edible, it does have a peculiar flavor to it that wasn't there originally, like when you store things together in the refrigerator and they start to smell like each other. It was also a little fizzy from the carbon dioxide. Like I said, edible but not that tasty. No bacteria or mold, though. Perfectly preserved.

We also tend to do political work at the institute. Trygve was a card-carrying member of the Libertarian Party of Boulder County (LPBC) when he lived in Nederland. I was the chairman of the LPBC for five years while I was doing the ice runs, and I would occasionally hold a political rally at the facility. The fame and notoriety of the FDG had been useful over the years for organizing political support and other things. Trygve always told me that Bredo was a libertarian, too. I've always said that we're all born libertarians and just learn to be different. I think that maybe we're all libertarians when we die, too.

One of the first events we held under the auspices of the institute was the Grave Digger's Lunch. The cryonic chamber had been collecting frost for years. I coordinated the lunch with an ice run in the summer so that there would be minimal ice left, and when I put it out to the e-mail list, I had four locals who were interested. Two couples came up that day, and we removed more than one hundred pounds of water ice from the chamber. After we filled up the chamber with ice again, everyone wanted to find out what it felt like to be Grandpa and hang out with him, so everyone climbed in one at a time and lay down for as long as they could stand it. We got some pictures, and a future Nederland town councilperson (and maybe a future mayor?) looked mighty good lying there.

Appendix

FAQ

Here are some frequently asked questions about the frozen dead guy, more or less in order of frequency asked. The answers are not always to be found within the rest of the book. The number one most frequently asked question?

Can you see him?
The technical answer is no. His remains are encased in a stainless steel, octagonal-shaped sarcophagus that is hermetically sealed and bound with steel bands. The sarcophagus is located in a plywood cryonic chamber that is insulated with six inches of foam and wood and has a hinged top. Only when the ice is low enough, like right before we throw more in, can you see even the sarcophagus. However, there is the only known (outside of the family) picture of a living Bredo Morstoel that hangs in the shed, above the chamber, as sort of a reminder of where we have been and of where we're heading.

How do you know he's really in there?
I have to admit, I cannot say with 100 percent assurance that he is in there, because I wasn't here for the beginning, when he was sealed in there. Trygve was. He's spent more than $250,000 putting together this property and storing his grandfather. He's spent more than $100,000 on the ice runs alone in seventeen years. That's a lot of money to waste on something that isn't

really there—especially as there wasn't even a hint of any fame back when Trygve started. Why wouldn't Bredo be in there? Where else would he be? Finally, I've seen a picture of Trygve, presumably at the cryonic preservation facility in California, sort of on one knee like a big game trophy hunter, holding open the partial lid of a silver octagonal casket/sarcophagus and looking at the camera and smiling. In the casket, you can see a very dead-looking visage that the caption said was Bredo right before they sealed him up. The casket looks exactly like the one in the shed.

Why do you do this?
The simple answer is that it's my job. My company, DTI Planetary Ecologists, originally took on Trygve as a client and maintained the facility in Nederland as a service to a client. Although we technically only get paid to do the ice delivery, we perform a number of services for the client, as we do for all of our out-of-town clients: property management, bill paying, record keeping and more things like that. The more complicated answer is that now that we've invested so much time and effort into it, it would be a shame to make a little screw-up and have it all be for nothing. In the early years, we wouldn't do a run unless I had the money in hand. Later, as the financing became more regular, we would occasionally do an ice run without actually receiving the money, as the responsibility of our actions overcame the fear of not getting paid.

Do you believe in cryonics and will you be joining him ever?
Surely you jest (sorry, Shirley)! As Grandpa said to the psychics, "Why would I want that decrepit old body back?" In my philosophy, your "soul" is immortal and just uses these fleshy "space suits" to interact on this plane of existence. To want to remain in any one space suit for more than your predetermined time is a waste of a good reincarnation. I personally think that we'd be better off working on building a body from scratch and transferring our psyche into that. Improve on reincarnation, so to speak. Preserving this "mortal coil," this "bit o' flesh," is a waste of resources and energy in my opinion… but I work for a client who believes in this, and my job is to do it as best as I can, with my client's mind in mind at all times.

FAQ

Are there other places where this is done and how do they differ from you?
Actually, there are at this writing (early 2011) a half-dozen storage facilities, five in the United States and one in Russia. There are another five or six companies that provide support services, like snatching your body when you die and taking it to the cryonic preservation facility or providing financial services. Alcor, American Cryonics society (ACS), Cryonics Institute (CI) and Trans Time all provide preservation services, as well as storage. Trans Time did up Bredo back in 1990. The IC Institute is the only facility that provides storage only, although we do provide limited preservation services for inanimates and small poikilotherms. Then, of course, there's the issue of dry ice v. liquid nitrogen (LN). We maintain that our cryogenic temperatures are adequate for preservation, while the "mainstream" facilities insist on LN, which is another one hundred degrees or so colder than dry ice, which is about one hundred degrees colder than regular ice.

Has this ever been done successfully before?
Not on a human long term. But there have been successes with freezing frogs and turtles for several months at a time, and when they were thawed out they appeared to suffer no damage. The main problem is how the freezing occurs. If it goes too slowly, it forms ice needles that puncture the cell walls and cause all of the juices to flow out. That's why things like vegetables and steaks get so soft and mushy when you thaw them out. All of the structures of the cells are compromised, and it becomes very flaccid. When the preservation at a cryonic facility is done correctly, the body is brought to a temperature just a smidgen shy of freezing for several hours to give the entire body time to equilibrate to the same temperature. Then it is "flash frozen" to try and freeze every cell in the body at the same time, without needle formation. The thickness of a human is the big factor. A frog or turtle has no cellular material farther than an inch from the outside when exposed to cryonic temperatures. It's at least six inches for some human parts, and the fat and bones tend to insulate and slow freezing even more. If we could "flash freeze" your entire body in a second or so, it would be a lot easier to reanimate you.

BIBLIOGRAPHY

Bergin, Edward, ed. *The Definitive Guide to Underground Humor: Quaint Quotes about Death, Funny Funeral Home Stories and Hilarious Headstone Epitaphs.* Westport, CT: Offbeat Publishing, 1996.

Geist, Bill. *Way Off the Road: Discovering the Peculiar Charms of Small Town America.* New York: Broadway Publishing, 2008.

Johnson, Larry. *Frozen: My Journey into the World of Cryonics, Deception, and Death.* New York: Vanguard Press, 2009.

Marquez, Ann. *Journey into Probate and Back.* Henderson, NV: Desert Muse Publishing, 2008.

Stockho, Pamalla. *One Too Many Frozen Dead Guys.* N.p.: Hawthorn Cottage Press, 2005.

ABOUT THE AUTHOR

Descended from politicians, carneys and renegade Scots, Bo Shaffer was born in Pennsylvania but moved all over the country as a child. His father was a lineman in the International Brotherhood of Electrical Workers (IBEW), and whenever he didn't like a job, he'd move on. Bo had lived in fifty different places by the time he was in middle school. After his family finally settled for a while in Upstate New York, Bo graduated high school and took off around the country again: college in New Orleans, Army Ranger School in Georgia, working on an oil rig in the Gulf, doing contract work for NASA in Houston, running a French crepe and omelet restaurant in La Jolla, surfing from K-38 to Steamers Lane, hand-crafting leather in Santa Cruz and eventually ending up at UC–Davis, where he worked as a vet surgical assistant while finishing his undergraduate degree.

After a couple more years bouncing across the country, he settled in Colorado and got his graduate degree in environmental biology. He was engaged to be married to his college sweetheart when she died in a terrible accident. Recovering in California with old friends, he met his soul mate, and they returned to Colorado six months later to settle down and start a business and a family. Bo worked as a licensed general contractor doing jobs for clients for several years until he decided to start his own environmental consulting and nontoxic construction company, Delta Tech Inc. (DTI Planetary Ecologists). One of DTI's first high-profile jobs was to be caretaker of the frozen dead guy.

About the Author

Eventually, Bo moved his family to a ranch in rural Boulder County, where he got into investment properties, politics and water. Chairman of the county Libertarian Party, Bo ran for several state and county elected positions, including county sheriff, where he got almost 30 percent of the vote. Bo was eventually elected to a local district government board, where he helps oversee an $85 million water district. Bo also sits on the board of CCTV54 and Channel 22, local access TV stations, where he also had a show called *Common Sense* for several years. Semiretired, Bo, his wife and their two children raise organic goats, chickens and eggs on their ranch. Bo and his wife will have their twenty-fifth anniversary the same year as the tenth anniversary of the festival.